WHEN THINGS
STICK

Untangling **Your Body From Old Patterns**

SUE CHOI

When Things Stick:
Untangling Your Body From Old Patterns

Published in the United States by Coherent Body Media

Copyright ©2023 Sue J. Choi

ISBN 979-8-9888118-0-0 (Paperback Edition)
ISBN 979-8-9888118-1-7 (eBook Edition)

First Paperback Edition: August 2023

Cover Design by Martin Vestgaard
Book Design by Femigraphix
Copy Editing by E. Lee Caleca

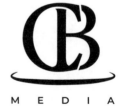

For Russ, who always believes in me.

"I could not recommend this book at a better time than now. We are building more understanding of how we learn through our embodied experiences and Untangling is a great guide on how to do this. As written in the book, 'when it comes to your body and perception, the experience needs to happen first.' See for yourself!"

—Dr. Stacy Barrows
Doctor of Physical Therapy, certified Feldenkrais® practitioner and PMA Pilates teacher, GCFP, NCPT~author and creator of the Smartroller™ tools to learn by

"There are so many reasons to read this book. It's full of resources and practical, tangible tools to transform your life. This book is a gift . . . and really it would make a great gift to those you care about in your life. As a dance educator, I find the information in Sue's book helpful to me professionally. I've been teaching various forms of movement over the past 25 years and find that Sue's clear and effective imagery is a great tool that helps my students access a deeper connection to their bodies. It is challenging when you teach a specific form as dancers are trying to copy shapes or style. This work gives them their own connection to the form, giving them a deep intuitive manner in which to connect to and master the work."

—Holly Rothschild
Dance Educator and Artistic Director of String Theory Harp and Bipedal Herd

"As someone who has professionally worked with people who are dealing with physical and emotional issues for over thirty years, I wish I had access to *When Things Stick: Untangling Your Body From Old Patterns* years ago. So many of my clients, consumers, and students could have benefitted from learning about this healing process.

I have personally been on a path trying different avenues for natural healing such as tai chi, yoga and physical therapy. Recently, I have had to do more invasive medical interventions. Nothing was giving me the full relief that I needed. *When Things Stick: Untangling Your Body From Old Patterns* helped me realize how much my body was stuck in old patterns. Written with compassion and insight, she gently guides us on a healing journey.

Personally, being able to find relief will help me to advise those who are seeking help outside of, or in addition to, traditional medicine to investigate this path.

This book is an invaluable resource for those seeking to untangle themselves and break free from old patterns that no longer serve them."

—Paige Lovitt
MS in Vocational Rehabilitation Counseling

"This book invites us into a life-changing, transformational journey: when we learn to listen to our body's guidance, we open to our bio-intelligent nature and our actions become coherent with what gives our lives meaning and purpose. Sue Choi is a trusted somatic guide who embodies her work and whom I deeply respect."

—Wendy LeBlanc-Arbuckle
Author of the forthcoming "BEYOND CORE: Your Inner Teacher's Guide Through Whole Body Relationships," to be published by Handspring Publishing in 2024

*Y*ou are about to join thousands of other people who have dramatically changed how they live in their bodies by following the instructions in this book. This book is an offering to start the changes that are possible and an invitation to go further if you choose to study directly with Sue. Here are just some of the outcomes from readers:

"I detached from my body at a very young age through the freeze response. I am now 65 and I'm still discovering patterns relating to the disembodied experience. When I first practiced the Sensing Posture I noticed the ringing in my ears stopped! Your book is helping me find the power to move forward. It has helped me see the ways in which I hold myself back due to fear that the environment isn't safe and something bad can happen to me if I wander beyond 'safety.'"—P.G.

"I have tried other somatic self therapies but for whatever reason, especially with the pelvis, I did not realize the tension my body was holding. THIS book unlocks and CONNECTS the entire body which I believe is the answer to much of my stuckness and extreme frustration of WHY I was still stuck. I am very, very appreciative!!"—K.C.

"What I have found is that my posture is being corrected. I really liked what you said about how trauma in childhood puts us into a certain posture. When you explained how the head, sacrum, and feet firmly on the floor all work together, I was happy to finally have it explained in a clear and precise manner. Since then I have often corrected my positioning whether I am sitting, standing or walking. I have noticed the biggest difference in my walking. I often find myself catering to the pain in my knees and legs, but when I walk upright like you showed us, I find it is so much easier to walk and with less pain. Just today I caught myself limping again and I adjusted my pelvis/sacrum and the change was immediate. I was able to walk without limping or pain. It was great!"—K.K.

"I felt the change, my knees and hips stopped hurting and emotionally I felt more open and strong."—K.B.

"I was stunned, laughing out loud and crying, when I hit the three keys and my body 'stood itself up.' That's what it felt like anyway. Weightless, effortless and with incredible balance. I felt like I was in a new body. Gorgeous feeling. Amazing. Who knew??"—M.C

"It was phenomenal to experience how my attitude limits me, because the resistance I have toward doing this stuff Is enormous. And I realized that when I come at it from a place of light and power it feels effortless."—J.K.

"It was like a small miracle took place. I realised for as long as I can remember I have never experienced proper breathing and have consequently been in a constant state of tension and panic. It's wonderful. AND—here's the kicker. I look younger. I have never felt so calm and serene in my life. This is the first time I've ever felt such a feeling of peace and connectedness. And I'm making better eating choices (WEIRD). I am making slower, more deliberate choices. I want my body to be well and nourished. I'm very excited by the amazingly quick and wonderful changes that are happening."—G.S.

Contact support@coherentbody.com to learn about working with Sue.

*"Life is never made unbearable by circumstances,
but only by lack of meaning and purpose."*
– Viktor Frankl

TABLE OF CONTENTS

INTRODUCTION

What's your body saying to you? The entire organization of the body is designed to broadcast messages that you can't ignore, whether you're conscious of them or not.

You know this already—you're not a beginner. You do yoga, meditation, tai chi—you know how much returning to your body calms your mind. But something's missing because you still find yourself trapped in old patterns and your tools for calm don't seem to work when you need them most.

In this book, you'll discover how you got stuck in the first place, why you're still stuck, and how to live in your body in a way that creates the changes you seek. Your body is your most intimate experience—no one knows it better than you. It has the clues to help you resolve difficulties that seem resistant to your conscious efforts.

The role your body plays in your emotions, behavior, and perceptions is too broad a topic to address fully in this little book. **So, my simple goal is to give you principles, skills, and tools to align your calm, inner experience with your actions so you can move forward with intention.**

How to Read This Book

You've picked up this book because you've been unable to move past old limitations that you've been struggling to overcome. *When Things Stick* will show you a novel way of understanding your body that will allow you to embody and integrate these new body tools so you can spontaneously use them as a natural part of your day in those challenging moments when you need them most. Because you're not a beginner, you might already know a lot, but you can't connect the dots. Or you might have a fragmented understanding of mind and body but continue to seek some way to bring all that information together.

If that's you, in this book you'll learn a specific framework that organizes your understanding of how sensations, emotions, and actions intersect. In order to apply these concepts to real life, you'll learn well-designed movements to create a new body vocabulary. Through this process, you'll also gain the skills you need to address and navigate your personal stress response patterns.

If that's not you, and you are new to mind-body practices, here's a caveat: this book might be a challenge to read. This book is not for beginners. Some terms and concepts are hard to grasp until you've had some practice and study in mind-body. That's because when it comes to your body and perception, the experience needs to happen first.

This book includes videos for you to practice moving your body in order to feel sensations. In that process, you will train yourself to observe your more subtle body signals.

If you have not had much mind-body experience, or if you just like to take action immediately, go to Part II and try the videos. But come back and read the rest to give context to what is happening in your body. I specifically wrote this book because context is what will transform the way you take action, how you pay attention, and how you integrate transformation into your daily life. Understanding the context is an essential part of the feedback loop from sensing into action and the spiral of learning as you move into more levels of depth.

It won't happen just by reading the book or by only doing the exercises. This is not something you'll get fully in one reading or one pass through the exercises. You must work it like a potter works the clay or a baker kneads the dough. It will happen over time as you reshape your body, feel your power, find your connections, and identify your new body changes as they contribute to your evolving concept of yourself.

Google Your Body

If you're old enough to remember the pre-Google search engine days, you remember how hard it was to retrieve useful information from the internet. Often, other search engines returned information that didn't truly meet your query. By organizing the world's information, Google made it universally accessible and useful. Likewise, when you organize your body, your body signals become accessible, and therefore useful.

Once you understand the signals, you'll discover your body is as powerful as your brain when it comes to solving problems so you can:

☞ Feel more physical comfort.

☞ Find more emotional calm.

☞ Get more clarity for taking action.

You will be able to unstick your body through your sensory system so you can resolve your persistent limitations.

Maybe you're not where you know you can be, and you feel the force of an invisible resistance that you can't name or shift.

Perhaps you can't overcome repeated patterns of conflict, either within yourself or with a loved one.

Or you might find yourself unexpectedly returning to old places that you thought you had conquered, and now you still feel stuck. What happened to all that practice?

Or maybe you've heard you need to be "more in your body" but just don't know what that means.

Starting the Process: How Does This Work?

To start the process, you'll go back to the basics of how you move. Standing and walking are the core actions that you'll improve with this approach. These simple acts, although pedestrian, contain a depth of unexamined riches when you discover how to consciously link the body that senses and the brain that creates meaning.

> **Client experience:**
>
> **Julia came to me with her experience going into her body to feel centered. She had a regular yoga and meditation practice, but she found herself feeling ungrounded and fragmented when she felt harassed by her neighbor. Something about this situation made her feel small and fragile, but in her mind, this was not who she was. This internal fragility was not what she identified with.**
>
> **In fact, at work, she felt powerful and in control. How could she feel strong outside of the environment where she held power? And how could she recover her personal, internal power when she needed it the most?**
>
> **This contrast between who Julia thought herself to be and what she was experiencing left her questioning herself, unable to reconcile the feelings that kept bubbling up.**

> *"I was initially in some deep trauma, and I would go so far as to say I was very depressed, but I'm not now. Your gentle approach to releasing trauma really works. My relationships and my confidence when I talk to people is like, 'This is how it is—this is it.' I'm not compromising myself in any manner. I feel like I'm in a power suit, I would say. I call it this power body—it's pretty exciting."*
>
> **What did she do? She practiced what I will teach you in this book. She learned to feel the stability of her body, which translated into a grounded feeling of power that she carried around everywhere, not just in her work environment, not just in her meditation practice. She was already experienced in noticing body sensations, but rather than swimming in the sensations, she had a process (one that you will learn in this book) for using them to move her forward when she felt stuck and to quickly feel centered and clear when she felt scattered.**

Before You Read Any Further, Try This in Your Body:

Stand with your feet 2–3 inches apart. Now, make the following move internally and imagine you are making it so no one can notice. Position your pelvis as if you are about to take a seat and send your shins forward at the same time. Remember, it's an internal shift, imperceptible to observers. Take at least 30 seconds to notice what happens. Take longer if you wish.

What changed for you? How did you feel in the whole of your body?

Now position your head to listen to the sounds around you and keep doing what you did above. Imagine you are waiting in line somewhere. Imagine people around you are impatient and stressed about waiting in line.

How do you feel? What changed now?

If you feel more grounded and settled, more spacious and open in the chest, or more relaxed in your shoulders, that's a good sign. (If not, try it with your eyes closed.) It's such a minor change to stand in this way, yet the change in your whole-body experience can be significant.

You position yourself according to the signals your body is giving you—the change it seeks. The body connects to the ground through the arches of the feet, which you activate by putting more weight into your shins while slightly changing the position of the pelvis.

Can you use the cues—shins, take a seat, listen—when you think of standing up straight? Can you imagine what would happen if you used these cues instead of bracing yourself in anticipation of something you fear/ dread/can't stand?

Now organize yourself as if you are listening from the front surface of your spine, deep inside you. Continue to reach your shins forward while you position yourself to take a seat within your pelvis. Let the sounds inside the room connect to the front of your spine—listen from the depths of that internal surface. Connect to the sounds outside the room with your ears.

What changed here?

When you organize your body to be touched by sound, both at the spinal level and at the level of awareness in how you position your eardrums to catch the sound, you feel what it means to be less defended in order to connect to the environment.

Simple internal adjustments on how to stand on your own two feet can generate palpable stability without the feeling of bracing yourself against an onslaught of environmental or emotional triggers. When you change that daily action of balancing on your feet, you feel trust in your own body.

Trust becomes an ambient feeling-state and gives you the resources to meet unexpected circumstances as they come up, those things that can throw you off. **When the body finds stability, the brain understands trust. You'll learn this through your Sensing Posture (see Chapter 4 for more on this).**

In this book, you'll also learn how to refine your walking. When you relearn the experience of what it means to move forward, you discover your capacity to metabolize old patterns that limit you. You do this by amplifying what is resourceful to you and using that to meet the challenges that hold you back. You alternate back and forth between what is resourceful to you and what challenges you. When the body walks, every step is an opportunity for change. **And when the body moves forward with ease, the brain opens to new perspectives (see Chapter 6 for more on this).**

These two acts—standing and walking—are potent but underrecognized agents of change. They are also deeply embedded in how you perceive and understand who you are. This entanglement all happened automatically through your development as you learned to organize your unwieldy baby body. It continued to happen as your hormones stoked the fires of action with emotional pokers. And it has been shaped through every action and response in your relationships.

This all happened without your deliberate attention. In this book, you'll learn that by going back to these basic human actions of standing and walking, you can peel away layers of the onion to form a new neutral shape. You can reclaim your body, form a new perspective, and generate your path forward using a process on which you can rely.

Where Does This Work Come From?

This body of work has evolved from three different streams of information.

First, it comes from understanding how to change a body through movement and through touching bodies. I've trained in multiple movement and bodywork modalities to help my clients resolve the most fundamental layers of their body problems.

Second, it integrates the visual and auditory systems as they apply to the coordination of the body. These two senses, along with balance, come together to converge perception through the organization of the entire body in the upright position. Vision and hearing are powerful resources that are typically not maximized. I've trained in vision and listening as they relate to how we organize our whole body.

Third, it comes from recognizing how movement and perception intersect with neuro-developmental models of the brain, emotions, and cognition, according to the way psychiatrists and neuroscientists view them. In the Recommended Further Reading section, you'll find a list of books you can read to dive deeper into their research.

Making sense—finding meaning—is what drives the whole-body and full-person process I'm presenting here. This may sound huge and overwhelming and ambitious, but if you start with the body first, it's actually concrete, easier than you might expect, and not merely the sum of its parts.

Before I started this work over two decades ago, when I felt stuck, swirling around in a depression that felt ancient and in a morass of sadness that had no origin I could name, I wanted to take action that mattered. I was pretty stuck and clinically depressed. The bottom of my tears felt endless, and I saw no way out. Talk therapy went nowhere and was disempowering. I was overflowing with feelings without direction, so I just shut them down. Without new skills, I felt like I was just treading water.

The system you'll learn here is a body-first approach that I've used not just once but over and over again to move past limitations—and so have my private clients. When the outlook for a solution is unclear, finding your center, strength, and ease will be a valuable resource and consistently instructive in how to move forward. My continued pursuit of a pared-down and integrated approach to relying on my body has led me here—to a system that simplifies the complexity of how our minds and bodies merge.

Although I started my way out of my crisis by using martial arts and yoga, I didn't truly learn yoga fully until I started to practice on my own. I was able to experience it quite differently when I began to explore and be guided by my own internal feedback instead of listening to instructions from someone teaching a room full of people. I'm seeking the same for you—that you can integrate the lessons into your daily behaviors and eventually become your own best teacher.

I've learned many other movement modalities since then and built sensing intelligence in my hands through bodywork. I've also learned about the whole-body impact of the auditory and visual systems and witnessed how trauma lives in the body. Through it all, the question of self-regulation was primary.

Self-Regulation Requires Body Tools

With this book, my hope is that you'll integrate these new body-based tools into your daily movement patterns so you can move past your limitations. You'll learn that the conversation you have with your body, using your senses and trained attention, contains wisdom and creativity you were not able to access before.

The changes you'll experience depend on what you are currently struggling with and what you already understand about your body. Read this, and after six months, see if you discover something different. You might find that you do. This work will be fluid; it will change naturally as you apply it because you will change in ways that might surprise you, ways that you could not see before because you were not yet open and your signals were not yet accessible, either to you or by you. It's an ongoing conversation with your body where you're listening and learning to speak its language.

A Trail Guide through This Book

To help you on this journey, this book includes:

☞ Videos that help you experience the concepts presented.

☞ Bonuses to help you get started as quickly and easily as possible.

☞ A reference list for further reading.

This book is meant to give you a fresh perspective on the body you know so well. It's a way to make peace with your body if you've been frustrated with it after having tried other things. Just using the videos can benefit you, but you'll get the biggest impact from the integration of these concepts into your daily life.

What you'll find in this book are concrete action steps plus the bigger context, because context matters for integration. When you understand how you create meaning through the body, you'll understand how to use your body to make changes in your thinking and actions.

Here's a trail guide of what you'll find in this book.

Part I: Determining if this work aligns with you.

☞ In Chapters 1 and 2, you'll go through some self-assessment to determine if this work aligns with your needs.

☞ In Chapter 3, you'll discover a reason you may not have considered that is keeping you stuck in the first place.

Part II: The practical application of the work.

☞ In Chapter 4, you'll learn how to stand on your own two feet through the Sensing Posture. You had a taste of it just now.

☞ In Chapter 5, you'll learn why your sensory system works when other approaches haven't.

☞ In Chapter 6, you'll learn how to metabolize old patterns and move forward with intention.

☞ In Chapter 7, you'll go over the impact of how these lessons converge within you.

You'll learn the tools that build the skills so you can follow the principles.

The Principles That Guide

☞ Stand on your own two feet
☞ Move forward with the whole of yourself

The Skills You Learn

☞ Find stability through your Sensing Posture
☞ Build trust in your capacity
☞ Internalize a template for action
☞ Be intentional in choosing

The Tools You Use

☞ Start with the videos in the book

I know starting something new can be a challenge, so if you want help getting the most from applying what you learn here, at the end of the book, you can learn more about my live online group coaching programs.

So, let's get going! I'm excited to introduce you to your new body.

Your body guide,

Sue

PART I:
BODY | MEANING | INTENTION

When you understand how the body intersects with how we form meaning, you can liberate yourself from blocks and integrate changes into a body that can tolerate and contain the whole of you. When your physical body is aligned with clarity of intention, the changes you desire can happen quickly and fully.

CHAPTER 1

Changes That Matter

*I*n these first two chapters, I invite you to determine if this approach is right for you. You'll hear how other people have transformed their lives. I offer these stories and the assessments at the end of each of these two chapters to help you determine if this material is right for you.

Client Experience: Kelly's Journey to Self-Trust

"I realize that I love my life! I'm so happy."

Nothing's changed in Kelly's situation except her internal experience of her body and how that impacts her relationships. She still lives where she lives, with her extended family, and has all the same responsibilities. Yet this inner shift allowed her to take actions that transformed the dynamics in her relationships.

Dramatic life changes had left Kelly in deep grief, adrift, struggling to adjust to living with extended family.

"I felt like an intruder in my own home, constantly trying not to annoy anyone, struggling for acceptance, inclusion. I recognized these familiar themes from childhood, but still felt stuck in a

repeating pattern. In addition, I felt physically fragile, unsure of my balance, wary of stairs and uneven terrain after several falls."

Despite decades of personal development and training, it was working through her body for the purpose of clarity and power that gave her the shifts in her actions that she'd been desperate to find.

"This way of relating to my body and the world around me literally put ground under my feet. Most surprising of all, walking itself has become a joy. A completely different experience. Just walking through the house, I feel like I am gliding; it is that free feeling, like ice skating, like dancing. Even the way the ground feels against my feet feels so good. So much more contact, like my feet are kissing the ground now."

And with that, her sense of herself began to change. She began to realize that her spaciness, the poor sense of balance that kept her from riding bikes, and her clumsiness were actually just avoidant strategies learned during the painful circumstances she'd grown up in—a withdrawal from being in her body. As she changed her relationship with the ground and with the physical world, she started recognizing changes in her relationships as well.

"Sounds crazy, but instead of walking on eggshells around other people, I started to feel myself actually getting energy and confidence from the way my feet contact the ground, the way I was walking. And I started noticing changes in my home life. As I interacted with family members from that calmer, more confident place, our relationships have blossomed, deepened. So much richer and more enjoyable. Now the challenges are just

> **challenges, things that (sooner or later) help me grow, not over-whelming things that break me or threaten my survival."**
>
> **So, in fact, everything's changed.**

What You Can Expect

You can learn this, too. You'll look at posture and walking in a fundamentally new way. You'll discover how organizing the gravitational force in your body gives you power, how listening with the whole of yourself gives you emotional connection, and how using your visual system the way it was designed to function gives you cognitive clarity. You'll learn that you can choose the story you tell yourself once you know the language your body speaks.

1. **Sensing Posture**—You'll learn how to experience what I call your Sensing Posture to feel more connected, more expansive, more stable, and more powerful. By focusing on the sensory experience of your body, you'll discover how to think of it as something you feel from the inside and how to generate feelings of wholeness and power, which lowers defensiveness. This changes how you experience your body on a visceral level.

2. **Walking pattern and resolution process**—I'll teach you one process of recovery that is rooted in a deeply human function: your walking pattern. You'll learn to leverage the organization of walking to recognize your inherent resilience. This is not the type of resilience you gain through boot camp; it's not about going to extremes to test your will. Instead, it's training your perception to identify the polarities inside of you and facilitate how these polarities organically resolve. You have within you the template to move forward, to unstick yourself by metabolizing old patterns that get in your way. It's there, and you only need to access it.

3. **Attention and perception training to increase capacity**—Third, you'll discover how to translate the language in your sensory body to meet more complex situations.

Client Experience: Jade's Journey to Better Self-Regulation

Jade's work colleagues are no longer afraid of her. They go to her to help mediate disagreements, something that was unthinkable a year earlier when they considered her prickly. Her supervisor now feels he can confide in her because she is not reactive, and her colleagues and subordinates feel like she truly hears their needs.

"After many years learning to communicate and be a great listener, training in mediation and crisis de-escalation, I noted in moments that an old and well-established pattern was still entrenched in my being—one of perceiving triggering situations through a filter of 'he/she is an asshole' or 'this situation is unfair.' I perceived the pain and discomfort I always felt in these situations as caused by 'them' or 'the situation.' It was never about me or where I was coming from."

Jade always had incredible skills to navigate difficult conversations, but those skills used to abandon her when she found herself caught in other people's arguments. When the people around her were acting out, she used to get angry with everyone and just disengaged. It was her strategy for creating boundaries that kept her safe. She knew this was not how she wanted to behave, and she knew where it came from. But despite understanding why she was triggered, she couldn't respond and use her skills in the way she wanted to.

"While feeling unseen and unappreciated, knowing that my intentions were to support and nurture, I also was unaware that I was not aligned with my intention, and this made the people I supervised feel stressed, criticized, and oppressed rather than supported and enriched.

Seeking the calmness and ability to be truly supportive to all of my coworkers, I focused on being accountable for my own internal process: to stop looking for what others were doing wrong to trigger me and piss me off. At one point, when triggered and angry, I used the tools you taught and focused on what happened inside, noticing, okay, I am triggered. I'm really angry. I let myself acknowledge and feel it. Then I noted my clear intention to not stay stuck in it. I committed to it and used the resolution tool to help me in that commitment."

Now she has a new capacity to be calm in herself when she needs it most. She doesn't need to escape in order to center herself and no longer blames external people or events for her reactions because she has the skills to find her center using intention. She can do this in the moment and navigate the uncomfortable without abandoning herself. She no longer feels that same frustration with others because she has internal space that enables her to listen with the whole of herself.

"I feel a new capacity for calm, to remain in or return to centered groundedness. I have an increased feeling of internal space and greater ability to listen with the whole of myself. I am increasingly able to see old patterns without the former level of criticism and judgment, and therefore I'm more motivated and able to move forward in balance and health."

What You Can Expect

In your daily life, what matters most is how you respond and make meaning out of the life you are living. That changes everything and doesn't require the need to run away or quit everything you know.

Many people quietly suffer and don't have the courage to investigate how things can be different. But that's not you. You're reading this because you have been asking the questions and feeling disappointed again and again that the answers you find are limited in their explanation, in their solutions, and in their impact. You've spent more than a good part of your life yearning to understand.

In this book and accompanying videos, you will find a way to connect your feelings into a framework that supports meaningful action in your life, the type of actions that move you forward.

1. **Perception**—You'll learn to change your perception of the world around you and the events that take place in your life.

2. **Insight**—You'll be able to *read* and understand signals that your body sends you so you can act on them appropriately.

3. **Empowerment**—You will no longer be a victim of your circumstances but instead see the opportunity for your intentional participation.

Client Experience: Bianca's Journey to More Energy and Youthfulness

Bianca feels in charge of herself in a brand-new way. She feels like she's dancing with her body instead of lugging it around. For someone who has spent a lifetime feeling off-center, she now feels childlike in the playful joy she gets in how she can move.

19

"For me, it's very important to have these moves as part of my repertoire that I can drop into, even if for three minutes; I can change my whole-body climate by running through these moves. Just doing them connects every part of my body and releases every part of my body."

She's no beginner when it comes to her body. She's tried everything she could to relieve her chronic pain from scoliosis. She's trained professionally to help others improve their posture. She's traveled to Africa to study dance.

"I thought I knew a lot about the body, but I'm finding out there is so much I didn't know. This goes so much deeper than I expected."

This process has opened her up to more mastery over her own movement, recovery, and ability to avert disabling downward spirals when she has a fall, gets a tweak in her knee, or feels her body act up.

The fact that she can feel light continues to surprise and delight her while giving her confidence that impresses her grown children. Overall, this new way of being in her body has increased her available energy since she is no longer fighting or over managing it all day long. Her body can keep up with her youthful spirit.

What You Can Expect

When you meet your body's needs in the way it craves, there's a palpable joy that comes through in your daily experience of it. This quality is beyond functional, and it will naturally draw you into changing your movement habits—not because you have to, but because you desire it and because it feels good to do so. You will want to move differently because it's a pleasure, not a chore. You'll find the time to pay attention in a new way because:

1. The changes are very quick.
2. The changes evolve and continue to build on themselves.
3. The new way of being in your body becomes integrated into your normal daily life.

Self-Assessment: Is Your Body Ready to Do This Work?

This approach is body first. That means there is a minimum level of physical fitness required to get the most out of this. It doesn't mean you can't benefit from what you'll learn here, but it does mean you may be limited in ways that can frustrate your experience of how I teach these concepts. So let's make sure that the videos that accompany this book are right for you.

Respond to each question below.

	Yes	No
Do you need asssistance to move up and down from a chair?		
Do you get out of breath after walking outside for 30 minutes?		
Are you dealing with a new (less than 6 months) pain that is impeding your daily function?		
Are you currently going through medical treatment that alters your capacity to work?		
Have you been diagnosed with a progressive movement disorder (Parkinson's, ataxia, dystonia, dyskinesia)?		
Do you have an unresolved vestibular disorder?		
Do you have a psychiatric diagnosis that you are trying to manage without psychotherapeutic help?		

If you answered "No" to all of the questions, then you qualify.

This approach is predicated on experiencing sensory signals in a new way.

If you answered "Yes" to any of these questions, this book is not oriented to your current altered sensory condition or movement limitation. If that's you, you're better off coming back to this work once you've stabilized your sensory body experience, have gained enough strength to pass this assessment, or have the full support you might need as you go through this work.

As a guideline, that means once you have learned the characteristics of your pain condition by working with in-person help for more than four months, or you are recovered from your medical treatment, or if you have been with your degenerative condition for over two years, or have a therapeutic relationship with a personal guide, you can most likely try this work. But be sure to consult with your doctor to see if you are cleared to exercise without supervision.

If you have an unresolved vestibular disorder, this work is not appropriate for you at this time, although you can still benefit from understanding how body, meaning, and thinking converge from the perspective of posture and walking.

To Summarize . . .

You'll learn how to use your body in what I call your Sensing Posture to feel whole and stable. You'll learn how to resolve old patterns and move ahead through the nuances in your walking system, and you'll learn how these two things can alter how you are able to perceive and think.

These changes are palpable, powerfully transformative, and practical. And yes, you'll feel great in your body as well.

CHAPTER 2

Smart Brain, Elusive Body?

*Y*ou've read a lot and learned a lot about the mind and body over the course of your journey, but you're still struggling. You're smart, so why is this so hard? Trying to grasp your internal experience and understand impulses that trigger emotions is sort of like a hand trying to grasp itself. You are fully immersed in your experience, so how do you get some perspective without disconnecting from your body experience? How do you meet yourself when you ARE yourself? You know the value of *being in your body*, yet the changes don't last. In this chapter, I'm going to cover some common struggles that I hear and why you might have those struggles. (In Chapter 3, I reveal the underlying energy-conservation bias that might additionally be keeping you where you are.)

Common Struggles

Here are common struggles that clients have grappled with before working with me. I'll explain how my framework was designed to address these problems.

Lucinda spent decades trying to understand her body because it was intolerable to be still in it. It asked to be stretched, to be adjusted, to be something other than what it was. As a successful executive with a master's degree, she couldn't think her way out of this struggle she'd waged every day since high school. The struggle had caught up with her, and she felt like she was on the losing end.

Julie, on the other hand, always felt fine. Everything was fine. She never complained, nor did her body. Until it really complained, and breast cancer took her on a long journey to reconnect to the unheard messages from her body—the deep signals of suffering she did not know how to hear. The diagnosis made her suddenly realize that her body was a stranger to her. She did not even know how to have a relationship with it. She was forced into a crash course to learn about her body. A decade later, she eats well, gets regular exercise, and meditates but still feels the toll that stress takes on her whole system. She thought she was doing all the right things and was frustrated that she felt more fragile than ever.

Sam takes care of her body and likes to work out. She likes to feel healthy and to be active. A series of injuries sidelined her, making her feel like she was devolving into old age. But she felt that forty-five years old was a bit too young to surrender. She wondered, "How can I trust that what I'm doing for my body is actually helping me?" Sidelined by injuries, she modified her exercise but didn't get the mental relief that she used to get when she was more active. A recent autoimmune diagnosis made her wonder why she was falling apart, and she began looking for new ways to manage her stress more holistically.

If you're feeling frustrated because you can't use your brain to figure out your body, what you'll learn here will open your eyes to the connections that make you feel whole.

If any of the following thoughts apply to you, then the solutions you'll find here are exactly what you've been seeking.

Why Isn't What I'm Doing Working?

People who get the most out of this work already have some (and often quite a bit of) experience working in their bodies to impact their minds. So that means the focus is on paying attention to how you feel as you work with your body. Despite all the work, though, you may still struggle with the emotional turmoil that takes you out of feeling your best for days, or weeks, or even months at a time. You may still feel like you're limiting yourself in ways you can't understand.

If this is you, then you know you can no longer band-aid the problem. It's not because you didn't try hard enough. It's because understanding the physical, mental, and emotional connection is a big body of work. You've probably learned pieces of it, but it still feels like a fragmented under-standing that doesn't seem to come together into a coherent whole.

Your practices fall short because you have no global approach for ongoing improvement or integration of changes into your daily life. Isolated changes that happen irregularly can't make the impact that you need to get over your biggest blocks.

What you'll learn here is designed to change ordinary, daily body move-ments that collectively impact you more than any class. By placing em-phasis on integrating the upright body, along with the visual and audi-tory systems, you'll learn how to work on multiple levels to make global whole-person changes.

I Can't Find the Time for Self-Care. It's Another Thing to Add to My To-Do List.

Perhaps you don't have a method to integrate the changes for self-care into your daily life. Do you feel great for 30 minutes after a class, massage, therapy, or other process but revert quickly to the familiar patterns when you're around other people? That's because the changes you experience in those contrived situations don't translate back into your day-in-day-out experience.

What is your ultimate goal in self-care? Is it just keeping your head above water? Are you ready to learn a way to move forward so you don't repeat your old dysfunctional patterns? First, you need the principles so you have a framework for insight. Simple tricks are not solutions. The magic solution isn't one muscle, one nerve, or one hack. Those were your starting points. **Tricks don't offer enduring insight that builds your proficiency.** They are stop-gap measures.

Instead, you can learn the principles that link the systems of your vision, hearing, and balance in a way that makes sense to your upright human body. You'll feel the changes immediately, directly, and eventually in your natural resting state. Because the intention of what you'll learn here is integration.

I Can't Always Make Sense of What I'm Feeling

Your human brain uses sensory input to create meaning. We are literally making sense of our experience down to the level of the neuron. In 2005, physicist, neuroscientist, and memory researcher Rodrigo Quian Quiroga published a paper in *Nature*[1] about large neurons he called concept neurons that store meaningful concepts.

This is a powerful discovery. It means that at the level of the building blocks of our nervous system, we are designed to create meaning. You are

---

1 Quiroga, R., et al. (2005). "Invariant visual representation by single neurons in the human brain." *Nature* 435, 1102–1107. https://doi.org/10.1038/nature03687

a meaning-making system. You are designed to make sense of your environment and your internal responses.

These concept neurons are programmable and changeable. You are bombarded every single day by thousands of sounds, images, interactions, surprises, and challenges. What do you remember? What stays with you and impacts you the most depends on what you give attention to.

When you learn to pay attention to the palpable sensory signals of stability, connection, and power, you truly *come to your senses*. As you get skilled in this process of intentionally encoding to metabolize what is stuck, you'll observe the power you can have over your narrative.

Paying attention to what you sense, being able to discriminate the nuances of that perception, and contextualizing the sensations into meaning is a learned skill set. I find that many people who say they cannot feel their body actually can do so when given the right framework and coaching. Once you gain that skill set, your capacity to perceive with trust, acceptance, and discrimination improves.

I Feel Disconnected from My Body

We are built to connect. Early bonding imprints our personal story of survival. A baby cannot survive without bonding with a caregiver because she can't fend for herself. But in phases, we also learn how to become independent. A baby becomes aware of herself as she separates from her primary caregiver. A toddler learns to stand on her own two feet. A young child fully develops intrinsic spinal muscles to activate her spine and discover her core. A young adult finally develops a fully mature prefrontal cortex to imagine long-term consequences.

What arises to replace that original reliance on the caregiver? You learn to activate that system in the Sensing Posture (Chapter 4). You truly learn to stand on your own two feet with security.

However, loads of things can go wrong in this process. If you've experienced insecure caregiving, a connection might look like neediness. Or if you've experienced abusive caregiving, a connection might look like dependency on destructive people or behaviors. Or, through early patterns of neglect, learned helplessness might be your pattern.

A distortion or defensiveness in body perception can form from past dysfunctional associations. **But you can feed new signals into your body when you learn to connect with intention to neutral and reliable forces—the gravitational field, light, and sound waves.** By doing this, you're starting from the body intelligence that has evolved over hundreds of thousands of years to support you. You can access a deeper human system intelligence instead of working from your personal thinking intelligence.

When that happens, you can stop compulsively correcting your body, like Lucinda, who discovered the capacity to find a stillness that is more powerful than any stretching routine.

Or you'll discover your personal power, like Julie, who discovered that managing stress is not about what she does but how she connects to the wholeness of how she feels.

Or you can lean into a framework to skillfully dive into the parts of your history that were previously too triggering to unpack. With this approach, already-healthy Sam felt the internal experience of a deeper health that created richer connections with the people in her life.

Are You Ready to Connect the Dots?

In this system, you'll relearn the things you already do on a normal day: standing and walking, listening and seeing. The depth of transformation you can experience by changing these things is a treasure trove of opportunities to make lasting changes and move forward, not merely tread water. By improving what you already do, you've built self-care into your essential movement patterns. Moving in your body in a skilled way encodes reliable messages that build trust in the stability of your body.

The principles of the body experience explained in this book are rooted in the most updated understanding of the human brain and body. Without resorting to myths or a belief system that is not in your culture, you can learn to reliably experience, through body explanations, what some refer to as *chi*.

There are enough specific skills you can learn in your own body that don't require decades of training under masters. You'll feel changes immediately. However, they do require a willingness to explore some concepts in a way that demands a fresh way of doing mundane things.

Self-Assessment: The Signs That This Approach Can Help

In addition to the statements I described, do any of the following sound like things you often think or say? Check all that apply.

I have to do it all by myself. No one helps.	
Never mind, I won't ask for help. I'll just do it.	
I need to fix this first, or to get over this, or to heal myself before I can *do what I would love to do instead*.	
I just need to make myself do X more, and I'll be fine.	
I never have time for myself.	
I can't seem to do what I planned to do.	
I want to make sure someone else doesn't get hurt—I can handle it.	

If you checked two or more items, you might have deleted yourself from your own story, have learned to disconnect from an innate trust in your body, or have become fragmented away from your experience of wholeness. This work will help you work out these concepts within the body to get beyond the thought patterns that are ultimately limiting you.

To Summarize . . .

The chronic limitations you are experiencing in your body right now have complex origins. Because you've been living with them for a while, they have become a part of your sense of self. You can start to dismantle these patterns when you start with this fresh perspective on how to just be in your body.

But you need a global strategy to change deep patterns. You can now investigate standing and walking as insightful actions that you take all the time, and those that your body has evolved to do well. You can harness that evolutionary body intelligence. When you do this, the integration of deep changes flows into your normal life.

CHAPTER 3

Is Your Brain Keeping You Stuck?

*I*n this chapter, we'll examine why you're stuck. I'm suggesting you might be stuck because that's just the energy-conservation bias of your brain.

The Blind Spot in Your Mind-Body Journey

Your body operates in the present moment, and you can amplify that moment using a sensing process. Your thinking brain can go into the past and imagine the future because it is capable of conscious creation. Your body gives signals of present-moment status that your brain then uses to direct action.

The sensing body has a need for connection. It's a meaning-making experience directed by the impulse to make connections: connection for survival, connection for safety, connection for belonging. The brain has a need to keep the lights on. It's highly sensitive to making the best use of your resources.

I'm suggesting that your sensory impulse for meaningful connection is trapped by the brain's energy-saving bias. This might be why it's so hard for you to move past your old patterns.

Meaning and Personalized Context

When we were babies learning about the world, the impulse for connection automatically created meaning. As our baby selves learned through interactions with the environment, emotions were automatically encoded to define those associations. For example, someone verbally abused by an early caregiver might develop feelings of low self-worth as a natural bonded state. This happens automatically without conscious participation because the brain remembers that experience and how it made this person *feel at a time when she couldn't consciously assess the impact it had on her*. The impulse for connection and the need for survival created a unified experience equating survival with an abusive relationship.

In order to unwind the meaning of patterned experiences, you must deliberately deconstruct beliefs by doing 2 things:

- ☞ Sense a new foundation of support and connection.
- ☞ Amplify resourceful experiences.

You'll learn to create a new sensing foundation in Chapter 4 and to amplify your resources in Chapter 6.

Your brain organizes meaning automatically. But once you understand how to do it, you can bring conscious attention and your embodied skills to shape your personal narrative—to live with intention. It's a thrilling and satisfying way to approach life. You will be present in your body, deliberate in where you direct your attention, and intentional in your actions. In fact, the alignment of your intention with your actions will feel satisfying because you'll fit into the patterns of your conscious choosing instead of your past unresolved struggles.

Energy-Conservation Bias

There is a process within you that is not concerned with your well-being. It's not intentionally sabotaging you. It just has a very practical purpose that requires a plan in order to overcome this bias. I'm talking about the brain's impulse to manage the body's energy. This process is the energy conservation bias in your brain which happens on two levels. Your brain seeks to conserve energy through homeostasis (internal set point balance) and pattern recognition.

Homeostasis: A Drive for Balance

Neuroanatomist Bud Craig located a very specific pathway of sensory signaling that goes into a deep section of the brain called the insular cortex. Sensations that go into this part of the brain from the body signal things like thirst, hunger, sleepiness, temperature, and pain. These sensations are designed to move you toward behaviors that help the brain maintain homeostasis. They get interpreted by the brain and form conscious meaning in the anterior cingulate cortex. Craig posits that this sensory perception is the seat of conscious thinking because it processes internal signals of our body's balanced regulation. These are the bottom-up signals that help shape our beliefs about ourselves, our behaviors, and our actions.

The insular cortex is your *inner feeling* brain and wants to keep your physiology balanced to conserve energy. You cannot stop this fundamental regulatory function, but if you disconnect from the signals, you deny your body's conversation with you. This self-denial is rooted in disconnection. Anorexia is an extreme form of this denial of homeostatic listening, but it can happen in more subtle ways as well. For example, you lose your appetite when you are in emotional distress or depressed.

But you can also make a conscious choice to overcome homeostatic signals. We commonly refer to this as mind over matter. Running a marathon is an example of persisting beyond serious protest from homeostatic brain function. Being able to intentionally overcome homeostasis is a skill. Disconnecting for survival, however, is due to a lack of skill in keeping basic connections. Once you have the skills to connect and stay connected, you can properly respond to the urges that keep you in balance.

Fundamentally, our feeling body signals energy conservation impulses that we can't listen to if we leave our bodies. What do I mean by this? I'll teach you more about staying in your body—feeling connected and whole—when I teach you the Sensing Posture in Chapter 4.

Pattern Recognition: Predicting the Future

The repeated patterns that frustrate you during a crisis are not surprising. Your brain is doing exactly what it's meant to do: predict what action to take based on recognizing patterns from prior experiences. In this way, it conserves energy by spending less time creating something new and less time course-correcting when it sticks to an old pattern.

That's the leading theory of brain function proposed by computational neuroscientist Karl Friston. The impulse of the brain in his model is to reduce prediction error. When you take action, it's based on your brain's prediction of outcome based on your mental model of the world.

Those repeated patterns that you can't seem to shake exist to save energy. Your current mental model of the world has been tested and updated by repeated trials of predicting outcomes. In times of crisis, your brain sticks to a rapid response it's honed over time. **Your brain is saving energy. It's not running in automatic mode in order to make you feel good about yourself.**

Changing Patterns Will Cost You

Right now, about 95% of your actions are automated, so making a conscious change to your status quo will require that you pay attention in a new way. In the same way your brain was trained by events to determine patterns, you can reteach it to believe something else, to react and predict in a new way. Changing your mental model and energy-conserving patterns can create great turmoil and will cost the brain a lot of energy, something it's not naturally willing to do.

The more experiences you have that confirm a pattern, the more bias you have toward repeating that pattern. That's why it requires a conscious and clear choice—intention—to overcome your biological resistance. The choice to make big changes to patterns that were formed from past experiences demands a lot of energy and requires permission. And that permission can only come from you, from your conscious observation and awareness of your internal states. Your narrative—the ideas you have about yourself, your mental model of the world—can be overcome through a resolution process that moves you forward. I explain that in Chapter 6.

Client Experience: Patricia's Journey of Recognizing How She Fed into Her Old Patterns

Patricia felt in a rut when it came to dysfunctional family relationships. But when she recognized her pattern in the moment, she was able to change her own response.

"My sister was having a difficult time and displaying old patterns of anger and bullying, and negative energy, triggering fears and a need for protection in me. I felt like I was leaving my body again. In the face of this challenge, I can see the old pattern of perceiv-

ing threat and danger, validating my need for protection and to feel safe, even though, as an adult now, I know there is no real danger. Using all that I've learned with you, I was able to reach inside myself for a feeling of stability to stay in my body instead. I felt my 3 Keys, mostly the Shin-Ankles, and how that put me more in my feet. I felt the front of my spine, like I was in the standing meditation, listening with all of my body."

It's easy to fall into old patterns. Patterns save you from doing the hard work of doing something new. Patterns conserve energy. But if you build the skill of learning how to feel stable and calm within yourself as your natural default stance, you won't need to escape your body—you will go deeper into it. And if you have a template of resolution that is built on the design of how your body moves forward, you are armed with a pattern of resilience. You can shift from an old destructive pattern of merely trying to survive into a more resilient pattern of movement and progress.

"Rather than investing in old patterns of self-protection and safety or attempting to control and correct a person or situation outside of myself, I was able to have a genuine conversation with her. I was able to establish a new pattern within me to find, like you say, connections and feeling purposeful movement."

By putting the brakes on her own disembodiment and instead going deeper into herself for feelings of connection, she interrupted the pattern of dysfunction.

"We had a conversation that dropped us into a new place. This is someone I never considered able to show empathy. She's always about herself, but by staying comfortable in myself instead of defensive, I could see her differently. It feels like I've been able to

integrate at a deeper level this understanding that the challenge of life is not to discern what is good and bad, right and wrong. It is to maintain balance while I allow myself to feel the ebbs and flows as they happen. I'm in awe of how I'm handling things. I feel such an increased ability to handle the challenging and hard stuff, more sure-footed and able to stay aligned and balanced in the face of life's storms."

To Summarize . . .

Your brain is trying to conserve energy, both to keep a homeostatic balance and to reduce recovery from error prediction. This bias works against change, so you are required to make clear and deliberate choices to change deeply entrenched patterns. But you can't just force it; you need to feel it. The experiences that created the old patterns continue to impact you because the patterns are energy efficient.

You can make a conscious choice to overcome this bias of energy conservation by diving into an enriched sensory organization to change your body first. When you use your sensations in this way, you'll feel a new reference to change your behavior. (See the Sensing Posture in Chapter 4).

Then, when you access your innate resolution process, you have a predictable framework to move forward. (See Moving Forward in Chapter 6).

Using what will eventually become your new embodied perspective, you'll get concrete body experiences through an internal reorganization that will ultimately support your intention to overcome the energy-conservation bias.

VIDEO LIBRARY

For your convenience, you can easily access all the videos in this book. Use your smartphone camera to scan the QR codes on this page. You'll find the QR codes within the chapters as well.

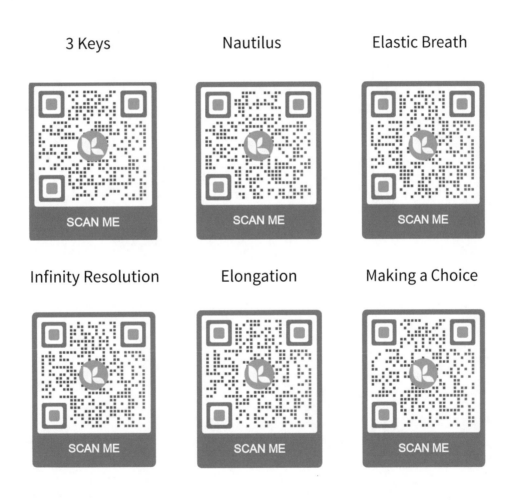

| 3 Keys | Nautilus | Elastic Breath |
| Infinity Resolution | Elongation | Making a Choice |

NOTE: These QR codes should take you directly to a video. There is nothing else for you to do. If you are asked for any personal or financial information, contact support@coherentbody.com.

To help you work through this book,
sign up here to receive bonus material:

https://www.coherentbody.com/when-things-stick-bonuses

PART II
SENSING AND MOVING FORWARD: PUTTING IT INTO PRACTICE

In this section, you'll put concepts into practice. First, you'll learn how to find your connections within yourself and to the forces outside of you, to help you feel whole and stable. You'll do this through your Sensing Posture (Steps A–C). Then you'll learn how to take action, which means reaching for resources first (Steps D–F). These two broad categories contain the step-by-step path to change your body and change your story.

CHAPTER 4

The Sensing Posture Is Your Path to Self-Regulation

The stories you tell yourself and the stories your body tells you should sync, but when they conflict, I'm suggesting the body wins. Let me explain how you can coax your body into a new story.

What is the Sensing Posture?

The basics of a body on Earth are one that all humans share: a long, flexible spine that sits on two long, comparatively inflexible legs attached to two small platforms we call feet. On top of this incredibly unstable structure is a heavy round head. Protecting that heavy head is vital because it carries some delicate tissue inside—a fall off the feet means great danger. The better your body can perform this task, the more your body can send signals of safety, power, and ease.

The conscious stories you tell yourself are stories of self-identity, belonging, and culture. These stories are personal and unique and help the brain make sense. When the brain can't make sense of what is happening, when you can't tolerate or process something in the moment, the experience lives on until you are ready to unpack it. In the meantime, per trauma expert Bessel Van der Kolk in his 2015 book, *The Body Keeps the Score*, you can't outrun it.

The burden of the human body tasked with staying comfortably upright is combined with the meaning-making part of your brain, which seeks signals to help build a cohesive story. The body story told by your body and the identity story told by your thinking brain together build a narrative that you live in every day. Can you change this deeply intertwined narrative? Yes, when you make the key connections in your system to give you new perspectives.

The Sensing Posture serves the purpose of optimally supporting the precious head in order to send you signals of safety, power, and ease.

How Does It Work?

Back in the day, you learned to walk but couldn't explain your needs in full sentences, couldn't regulate your toileting needs, and didn't know what it meant to navigate social norms. Initially, learning to stand and walk was a significant period of self-regulation, where you developed a level of conscious control over your body. This control took you forward into adulthood.

What if you went back to these essential actions of your human body— standing on your own two feet and moving ahead—to reimagine what it means to feel secure, to feel powerful, and to move forward with ease, the way your human system was designed to move. Relearning this as an adult is an act of reclamation.

When you organize your body from the Sensing Posture as an adult, you come home to your body with more wisdom and a richer context of conscious insight than you had when you were a drooling toddler, patching together a worldview before you could really have conversations. You can feel calm, confident, and optimistic in how you interact and connect with the world because you are deepening this self-regulatory triumph. This essential human act of self-trust establishes independence on the one hand, yet necessitates deep internal connections in order to keep it all together.

The sensory information of your upright body encodes the concepts of being grounded, feeling connected, and finding your center as the palpable baseline experience of your daily life. This is your Sensing Posture, and you will relate it to your personal story through pattern recognition, metabolizing old limitations, and conscious choice in how to move forward.

Three Steps to Access the Sensing Posture

Here are the steps to strip yourself back down to the ordinary body experience of humans so you can clearly witness the difference between your identity story and what is just a body on Earth.

The Sensing Posture is the first phase of changing your body story. In this stage, you are working with the nuts and bolts of posture: what a body needs to balance in a comfortable, effortless way. To give you an idea of what's to come, here's an overview of the 3 steps to your Sensing Posture:

Step A: Calm through internal connection.

Step B: Power without strain.

Step C: Ease through a body that breathes itself.

Step A: Calm through Internal Connection Using the 3 Keys

I've identified three key pivot points in your body that give you the experience of distributing tensional support throughout your body. There is a webbing called fascia that weaves through all your muscles and organs and wraps the bones. Using these pivot points is one way to address this system with one global gesture of squatting inside yourself.

You will learn to access the movements at the pivot points and what you need to change within yourself to get there. These movements contain everything you need to make a profound change in how you balance the weight centers in your body.

The 3 Keys

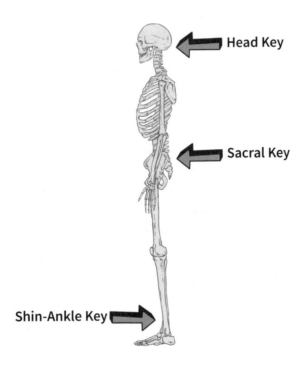

1. Head Key: the base of the skull.

2. Sacral Key: the sacrum, the triangular bone at the base of the spine between the two hip bones.

3. Shin-Ankle Key: the shin bones, just above your ankles and just inside the ridge on those bones.

You got a taste of that in the intro, where you took a seat, pushed your shins forward, and opened your ears to listen. This posture helps you position your head to activate the Head Key.

VIDEO: 3 KEYS

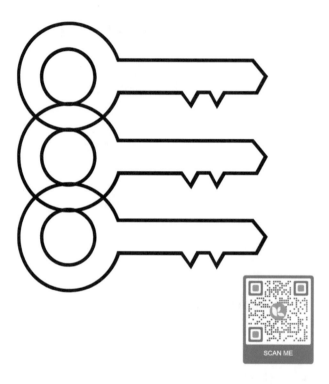

SCAN ME

Before reading further, take 10 minutes to watch the Introduction to the 3 Keys video. In it, I explain how the 3 Keys work and walk you through trying it out in your body. When you've tried it a few times, come back here for more context.

<u>WHAT IT IS IN THE BODY:</u> The 3 Keys are the **Head Key, the Sacral Key, and the Shin-Ankle Key.** This process will balance a tensional webbing in your body (called fascia) by reorganizing how weight is managed in your body through these key pivot points. The purpose of the 3 Keys is to give

you a quick way to distribute tension in your posture for balanced support, directing the weight of the body down through the bones. The 3 Keys make it possible for you to access your most effortless posture.

<u>THE MEANING YOUR BODY SENDS TO YOU WHEN YOU USE THIS:</u> This state of tensional balance communicates messages of support, wholeness, spaciousness, and balance.

More Details About the 3 Keys

The shin-ankles, when fully used, drive the weight of the whole body down into the arch of the foot and back into the inner heel, in order to access full use of your foot and the lower leg. Focus on moving weight into your shin-ankles to change the way you leverage your weight in every step. But to protect the knees from strain, you have to direct movement through your sacrum.

The shin-ankle is located on the shin, near the ankle, just to the inner side of the pointy front edge.

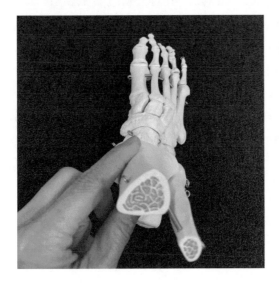 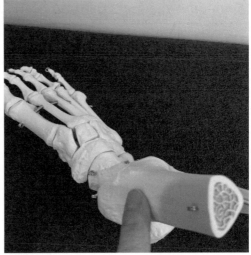

When you put weight into this point, it distributes the weight of your body down and back toward your inner heel.

This weight distribution into your foot stretches the plantar fascia and distributes weight through the arch of the foot.

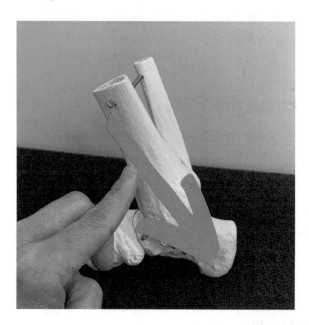

When you lock your knees, for example, the weight doesn't travel at this angle into the foot. Over time, this can lead to quite a bit of dysfunction, such as plantar fasciitis or lack of hinging at the ankle joint, which in turn leads to too much stress on your big toe joint.

The sacrum is a triangular bone that transmits weight from one side of your body to the other and is also the base of the spine.

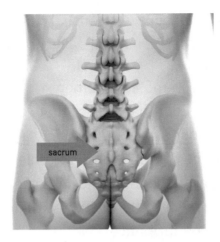

You might think of the pelvis as one big bowl, yet there is a subtle but powerful coordination that happens between the hip bones and the sacrum that makes all the difference in how you navigate the pull of gravity through your body. We'll discuss this more deeply when we talk about the Nautilus.

The base of the skull supports the weight of the head in a way that activates the global tone in your postural muscles. There are signaling receptors in those muscles that feed directly into the cerebellum, which organizes coordination and balance. Sometimes it's easier to access the Head Key if you imagine lifting your cheekbones slightly upwards so you can look off into the horizon.

What words would you use to describe your outcome?

This video shows an extreme movement you can make using the 3 Keys, but this is not the goal. Most people will get stuck trying this version due to limitations in the pelvis or spine, and many people will not be able to do this.

But here's the beauty of the concepts you're learning here: you can still learn how to access your internal connections by keeping these 3 Keys in mind. You don't have to perform

49

extreme moves in order to feel a difference. The most profound difference will happen in how you change normal daily movement patterns.

Much of what you'll find in most movement training comes from the extremes of performance. But what part of that training is most transferable to your body and your daily life? I would say it's not a physical skill in the context of extreme competition. Top athletes have been shown to demonstrate better proprioception and interoception. They experience their bodies with more precision to overcome their internal resistances so they can improve their performance.

Those refined discrimination skills are what you are learning here—the internal sensory vocabulary to meet yourself so you can improve your connections, both within yourself and to your environment. The benefits are practical as well as emotional.

Client Experience Using the 3 Keys

"After a long day of sightseeing, I had excruciating pain in the bottom of my left foot—excruciating. I hobbled my way from the car to the hotel, and I went to bed. I got up the next morning. My whole foot was swollen. I could hardly walk. I concentrated on the shin-ankle in that foot, and you know, within the half hour, I could walk without pain. And I did it by entirely transferring weight to that foot.

And when I did the shin-ankle transfer the way we did it in class, it opened a door, and the blood could get out of the foot. I healed myself by walking miles, by doing that thing, by weight bearing and concentrating on the Shin-Ankle in that foot. It was just remarkable. And it came back three days later, and I did a Shin-Ankle, and it went away."

"That whole thing changed my whole body, my torso alignment, my foot, and leg usage. So that was a stunning experience, and I walked miles every day in Washington.

I didn't have time to build bad patterns into my body from hobbling on that painful foot because I resolved it right away."

Activating the 3 Keys

You can activate these 3 Keys simultaneously in one of two ways: standing or seated. Eventually, going from one to the other will liberate the postural patterns that limit you. By training yourself to coordinate these 3 pivot points in those transitions, you direct movement through your fascial webbing with global impact.

Try it first in standing.

Place your feet 2–3 inches apart.

Turn on your Head Key by lifting your cheekbones or imagining a crease at the back base of the head.

Now take a small, tiny mini-squat as a way to activate your 3 Keys.

As you do this, reach your tailbone down and back as if you have a long dinosaur tail.

By activating the Keys simultaneously, just a little bit on each Key, you are coordinating these pivot points to generate a movement pattern that allows your skeletal system to support you.

Now try it again with your hands behind your head and your fingers interlaced at your Head Key.

NOTE: If this hand placement is difficult for you, place your fingertips on the base of your skull, behind the ear on each side. You can pivot on these points instead.

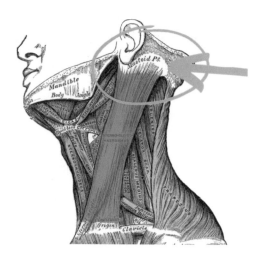

Attribution: Image: Gray385.png modified by Uwe Gille, Public domain, via Wikimedia Commons

Now try the mini-squat again.

Test it out a few more times.

Now try it in a seated position.

Start by sitting on a chair with your knees wider than your hips.

Sit so half the length of your thighs or more are off the seat.

Slide your feet back toward you so your knees are just over or beyond your toes.

Your hips should be slightly higher than your knees. If not, find a higher chair or use a towel to prop your seat up.

Place your hands at the Head Key or in the alternate position.

Shift your weight into your Shin-ankles as if you are about to stand up off the chair.

Send your dinosaur tail back at the same time.

Feel your chest lift up?

If not, come back after you've learned the Nautilus and give it another try. Just shifting your weight into your shin-ankles might reorganize your spine, relieve your back pain, and open up your chest.

Now try to stand up from the chair, putting weight into the shin-ankles, keeping your tailbone reaching back as the base of your head stretches away from the tailbone.

If you have to swing your head forward a lot in order to get off the chair, try sitting closer to the edge of the chair.

Try putting more weight into your Shin-ankles.

Make your knees track over your 4th toe.

For many people, that might mean spreading the thigh bones wider. Your knees should never hurt when doing this.

Walk around the room. What changes do you notice? How do your feet feel? And what about your back, chest, and shoulders?

3 Keys in Daily Life

You can use the 3 Keys as reference points during your day to help organize your body position and movement. Here are some suggestions on how you might use them throughout your day:

Feel the weight in your shin-ankles and reach your dinosaur tail when you:

☞ walk up and down stairs

☞ step off a curb

☞ get up off the floor

☞ climb steep terrain

Use Shin-Ankle and Nautilus to secure your lower body when lifting heavy objects.

Activate the Head Key when you:

☞ feel yourself slouching

☞ feel sleepy and want to stay alert

☞ feel shoulder pain

Use the Head Key when turning your head:

☞ Use the base of the skull on the same side to turn toward that side (i.e., use the RIGHT base of the skull when turning your head to the RIGHT).

Step B: Power without Strain Using the Nautilus

In the Sensing Posture, you find power by circulating the force of gravity through the skeletal structure using a concept I call the Nautilus.

The Nautilus is a way for you to harness the pull of gravity down through your bones and distribute it back up through the front surface of your spine. The Nautilus movement in the pelvis gives you access to the hydraulics within the diaphragms of your body by learning how to differentiate the action of the sacrum and your two ilia (two big bones we commonly call the hip bones).

By coordinating the sacrum and deep core muscles, you will access power with very little effort.

Gravity pulls you toward Earth, but you can harness its energy. This becomes your path to a power that is greater than your muscular strength. Instead of using your muscles to move you, you are accessing the internal mechanisms that generate the power. It's the difference between pushing the car to move it and pushing on the gas pedal. This step is about finding the gas pedal.

VIDEO: NAUTILUS

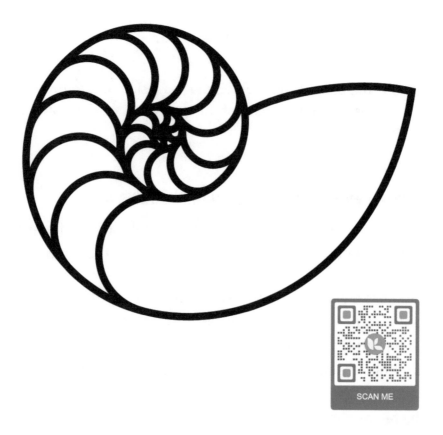

SCAN ME

Take five minutes to watch me explain the Nautilus concept. See if you can feel it as you go back to the 3 Keys. Then return here for more context.

<u>WHAT IT IS IN THE BODY:</u> The Nautilus helps you access differential movement in your pelvic girdle to redirect gravitational force up through the front of the spine, all the way up to the head, and back down the back into the feet.

<u>THE MEANING YOUR BODY SENDS TO YOU WHEN YOU USE THIS:</u> The Nautilus gives you access to feel your power without creating strain. This effortless power gives you confidence and stability.

More Details About the Nautilus

If you consider the shape of a nautilus, it is a rotation on itself that pulls inward. It's a consolidation. Often, we are taught core as a bracing or effortful action. When you find the Nautilus movements internal to you, it drives the larger movement without strain. If you think of the gears of a watch, the gears move the hands without displacing themselves. Similarly, the Nautilus moves within itself to create power for stability and an anchor for movement.

There are two places you can access this Nautilus movement: your <u>pubic bone</u> and <u>iliac crests</u>. I'll refer to them as the little nautilus and big nautilus. They both spin backward.

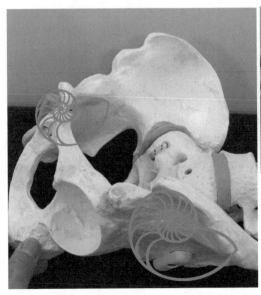
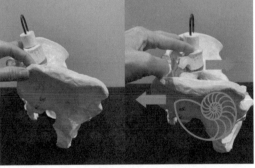

When you generate the nautilus movement, the contrasting movement of the backward spin and the forward tilt of the sacrum creates internal space for the spine to lengthen.

Regardless of your position or your spinal movement, the Nautilus spins backward. In opposition, imagine the upper part of the sacrum tilting slightly forward while the tailbone reaches back.

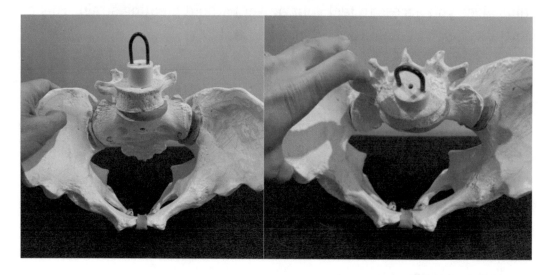

When you move the pelvis with the Nautilus movement while tilting your sacrum forward (or dragging your tailbone backward), you open your back pelvic floor. Can you feel what that does to your upper spine and chest?

There's a lot of patterning in the pelvis. Using the Nautilus to change the patterning from the inside while you're seated, on your back, or standing is like doing bodywork on yourself. Instead of stretching your back, experiment with using the power of the Nautilus movement to release what is tight. This gives you access to experience your power source from the deep front surface of your sacrum. In martial arts, they call this the *dan tien.*

The distinct movement of the Nautilus with the tilt of the sacrum creates a hydraulic circuit that moves up the deep front surface of your spine, and your arms will feel like they are being sucked down into their sockets. Note that the Nautilus always goes in the same direction, regardless of your body position and the direction of movement of your whole body.

After trying the video, what's your experience of your body as you stand and move around?

Client Experience Using the Nautilus

"Honestly, that's just the answer for me every time, right? More Nautilus. When I access the Nautilus, it connects everything for me. I feel that front line. I feel the whole-body connection. I feel secure and grounded. It still surprises me how simple that is."

"I hear your voice in my head when I feel myself slipping into old pain points. The other day when I felt that old hip thing happening again after I had family in town for a week, I decided to make the choice to work with more Nautilus in the last couple of days of the visit. Wow. Just wow. I could really stand my ground, and I felt like an adult for the first time in my life when I was speaking to my mother."

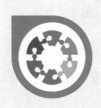

Activating the Nautilus

The 3 Keys help you with positional awareness to maximize skeletal support and balanced movement through the joints. The Nautilus helps you access intentional power by aligning your weight through the skeleton with gravity instead of fighting against it. It's like surfing—you ride the power that's bigger than you.

Try this first in a seated position.

Start by sitting on a chair with your knees wider than your hips.

Sit so half the length of your thighs or more are off the seat.

Slide your feet back toward you so your knees are just over your toes.

Place your hands on the top crest of your hip bones, holding them as you lean forward.

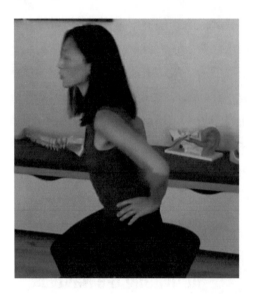

As you lean forward, reach your dinosaur tail down and back while spinning your big nautilus.

Try again and practice using your little nautilus as the engine that helps tilt you forward.

Make sure you feel weight go down into your shin-ankles.

Do you feel your collarbones lift and widen?

Now try it in standing.

Keep your hands on your hip bones.

Make sure you feel your shin-ankles.

As you move your big nautilus, be sure to keep your tailbone reaching down and back.

Now try another way.

Find your shin-ankles again.

Spin your little nautilus, making sure it is aligned under your head.

Spin your big nautilus.

What happens?

Do you feel your feet suctioning into the floor? Do you feel your chest open and lift?

Now let your arms hang. Spin your Nautilus

Can you feel your armpits suctioning your shoulder blades down?

If so, that's great—I call this the Nautilus circuit.

The Nautilus circuit goes up the deep front surface

of your spine and down the deep back and side surfaces of your spine.

That armpit/shoulder blade feeling indicates the circuit is fully connected.

If you can't feel it yet, don't worry.

Chances are the circuit is impeded somewhere near the diaphragm, and as your body changes, you will eventually find it.

Step C: Ease through a Body That Breathes Itself Using the Elastic Breath

Note: This may be the hardest thing to feel immediately, so learn the basics and know this will improve as your whole-body structure changes, particularly your upper chest and your pelvis.

The Elastic Breath is a way to access full nasal and diaphragmatic breathing using proper positioning of the tongue and full–body posture. Your tongue should rest in a relaxed and wide position against the roof of your mouth to support nasal breathing, full movement of your ribcage, and synchronization between the diaphragms of your pelvic floor and the base of the ribs.

Breathing is a complicated process and prone to many poor patterns. Breathwork training can be fraught with bad and dangerous instruction and has the potential to create dysfunctional habits. To limit acquired dysfunctional breathing patterns (which can happen by forcing a breathing style), the Elastic Breath is a concept that is tied to the whole-body experience of breathing.

VIDEO: ELASTIC BREATH

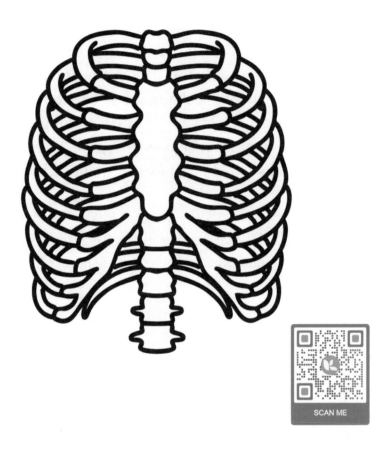

Watch the video to try this out on your own first. Ultimately you want to allow your body to breathe naturally. But we get trapped in our own limitations, and a poor breathing pattern is a big limitation. The concept of the Elastic Breath, like all the concepts you'll learn in this book, is a reference point, not something you perform to fix yourself. The intention here is to give you some key insights, and no matter what breathing training you might pursue, these insights are applicable.

Your breath is controlled in a few ways. Dr. Rosalba Courtney, osteopath and breathing expert, identifies the three dimensions of breathing: bio-chemical, biomechanical, and psycho-physiological. In the Elastic Breath, you follow the biochemical signaling with a biomechanical assist to open psycho-physiological possibility.

<u>WHAT IT IS IN THE BODY:</u> The Elastic Breath is the feeling of full-body breathing—from the depths and width of your sinuses down to your pelvic floor. Chronic poor breathing mechanics are common and create an in-flexible rib cage that is difficult to change with breathing mechanics alone. Postural organization from inner signals brings the breathing mechanics back into balance and gives you the feeling of inhabiting a body that is whole and stretchy.

<u>THE MEANING YOUR BODY SENDS TO YOU WHEN YOU USE THIS:</u> The mes-sage you feel from free and easy breathing is a signal of safety, calm, and effortless energy.

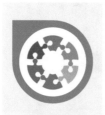

Combining Elastic Breath with the 3 Keys

Let's work with this in standing. Be aware of your 3 Keys.

Swallow and notice where your tongue rests when you do that. Let it magnetize to the roof of the mouth and spread wide. Feel an internal smile. Imagine that your tongue is on the floor of the sinuses and see if you can feel how it would move with your inhale.

You can also connect the concept of your tongue position as an extension of your Head Key. Together they create a platform to support the weight of your brain.

Now imagine the base of your pelvic floor is a diamond composed of two triangles.

tail bone

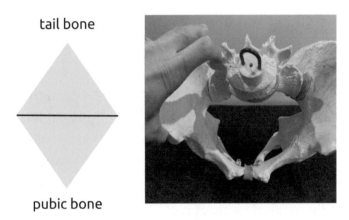

pubic bone

Feel the back triangle stretch out behind you by reaching your tailbone away from you. You can imagine your sacrum grows a long heavy dinosaur tail that drags back behind you. Make sure you keep weight in your shin-ankles while doing this.

When you inhale, feel the tongue widen and flatten, while the back pelvic floor triangle stretches back. When you exhale, both the tongue and pelvic floor dome upward. Can you feel them work in tandem?

Client Experience: Using the Elastic Breath

"This is such a different way to work with the breath. I get really anxious when I do breathwork, and this just feels different. It's easy and gentle. I use the tongue and Head Key on those days I have my long commute to work. I arrive feeling less frazzled, with more energy."

A Note If You Have Trouble Sensing Your Body

You may think you don't feel your body very well, but maybe you just haven't had the right training? It's usually just a matter of how you pay attention. You may have become biased to feel discomfort and ignore what feels great. Or you may have chronic pain that colors all your feeling with the color of pain. Or you may be highly skilled at disassociating.

What you're learning to feel here is all the normal signals of pleasure and joy to which you no longer pay attention. You are learning to direct your attention to what works, gives you pleasure, and excites you to reach out. This is a life-saving skill that can be cultivated.

For example, do you have a pet? How do you feel when you are stroking their fur? Where do you feel it? How would you describe the sensation?

- ☞ With volume (I feel expanded in the chest).
- ☞ With temperature (I feel warm in my face).
- ☞ With movement (I feel my shoulders relax).

What's your favorite song? Why is it your favorite?

- ☞ Does it evoke a memory?
- ☞ Do you feel yourself smiling?
- ☞ Do you feel yourself moving with the music?

You have many regularly occurring examples like this in your life. Subtle but essential, the capacity to focus your attention on how these moments of pleasure live inside you is your power to cultivate embodied resources that you can use to meet and neutralize difficulty.

Review These 3 Steps to Create Your Sensing Posture

Let's review what you've experienced so far. You are learning to stand on your own two feet, quite literally. Remember, the 3 Keys, the Nautilus, and the Elastic Breath give you access to the wholeness of your posture.

You can work with any of them on their own, but ultimately, you'll find the connection between the concepts. For example, can you feel your shin-ankles when you activate your Nautilus? Can you imagine how your Head Key and Nautilus work together to activate the front of your spine? Can you feel the platform that the tongue and Head Key make to support the brain?

Together the 3 Keys, the Nautilus, and the Elastic Breath create your Sensing Posture. The Sensing Posture activates the front surface of the spine, which is essentially our core. We're standing in our core. We are inhabiting a part of us that conducts gravity upward. And by conducting gravity upward, it anchors us to the floor in a new way. It's not just a balancing act; it's a deliberate act of presence that feels like the statement, "I'm here."

BONUS VIDEO: STANDING MEDITATION

To illustrate these points, here's a bonus video (36 minutes) of me taking a group through a standing meditation process and turning on the Sensing Posture. This video contains two standing meditation experiences as well as people sharing their outcomes. It's worth hearing other people's experiences because, in the end, we are all working with a body standing on Earth, and people have learned a lot from the experiences of others in these sessions.

Sensory Intelligence

When you begin operating from your Sensing Posture, you'll discover how smoothly things should have been working all along. It was always there; you just lost touch with it. More than muscles, bones, or nerves, the sensory system is the signaling system that activates everything else. It is, by design, highly adaptive. You'll discover self-organizing mechanisms you've been neglecting. It might feel like magic, energy, or *chi*, but I prefer to say it's just a body that is working as a whole all at once. You don't need to bathe it in mystery in order to organize it within you.

This essential version of your body has the evolutionary intelligence to operate this delicate and marvelous balancing act, all the while broadcasting the messages you've been needing: *I'm supported, I'm connected, I'm anchored, I'm whole, I'm at ease, I'm powerful.* You'll learn to feel those messages in your bones and tissues so the ideas in your conscious brain arise from material truth. You'll be able to discover, again and again, embodied wisdom that propels you toward your desires.

From decades of working with clients, here's what I know:

Working from this foundation will constitute a huge change in how you inhabit your body. But in order for it to integrate into your self-perception, you need more than the body approach. You need to understand how this new body relates to the emotional and thinking parts of yourself. This is why you'll learn this foundation along with the messages that it sends you —messages of support, power, and ease.

Continual new messages like these eventually create an identity that may feel very different from what you're used to. Or they may bring you a sense of déjà vu, of having been here before. And in fact, this is exactly what is happening. You are not inventing something new in yourself; you're rediscovering a less conflicted version of yourself. These persistent messages from the Sensing Posture will feed into a global self-perception of calm and clarity.

However, as I mentioned, lasting deep internal shifts in your body don't happen by just changing the body. You need a process to dismantle old patterns of self-perception so you can make new choices.

To Summarize...

The Sensing Posture gives you access to a deep level of perception without judgment, analysis, or personalization. It gives you access to the foundational messages of a resourceful body. Your Sensing Posture tells a story about your humanity. Body function and the meaning they signal are both necessary as you access your Sensing Posture, so be sure to recognize them as you go through movements. It's easy to fall into a do-ten-reps mode when moving the body, but don't do that. These movements are designed to be exploratory. Think of them as a way to do bodywork on yourself, and sit with the question of how the associated meaning lives in your body.

Feeling connected and powerful in your body allows you to lower your defenses, and dismantle the walls we put up to protect ourselves. Your Sensing Posture allows you to feel your internal landscape.

CHAPTER 5

An Entirely New Approach Requires Thinking Differently

I'm going to spend some more time here talking about how sensations can change your body experience because, in my experience working with clients, this takes a while to really absorb. The reason it takes a while is that this shift requires a fundamental change in how you relate to your own body from a *doing* body to a *feeling* body. That's not going to change in a single experience. Like any new relationship, it is going to evolve, and it requires active conversations.

Fundamental Change

Do you remember the first time you recognized how you could calm yourself when you felt overwhelmed by emotion, stress, or uncertainty? How old were you? What was it? How else have you learned to use your body to be in charge of yourself?

By this point in your life, you already know that you can take a deep breath to shift your emotional state, that stretching feels good to feel more spacious, and that walking it off to problem-solve is helpful. You might know that certain auditory assists help you focus for work (headphones, classical music, certain background sounds like office noises), and other auditory assists help you focus for calm (nature sounds, white noise, Tibetan bowls). If you've had panic attacks, you might know that looking for and naming colors helps bring you back into your body.

You already know a lot about your body, your senses, and how to manage them to impact your state of mind. So how is this different? Most somatic approaches don't address how the body's experiences come together to tell the narrative of your life and shape your identity. We have an intimate perspective of ourselves that no one else can fully know. You yourself may have hints of things about yourself that you can't quite parse out consciously, yet they show up in your actions and behaviors in ways you might regret or in ways that don't fully express how you want to show up in the world.

You are immersed in your story, and it has many dimensions and a lot of complexity. Like any story that is well-written, the journey is engaging and surprising but ultimately satisfying because it moves forward. You are writing your story while living it. Is the journey satisfying? Can you find the connections that make a storyline? Is your story interesting to you? Can you edit and un-fragment your life experience into a narrative that engages your interest?

If you are not consciously and intentionally creating your own meaning from your experience, it will be written for you. Imagine a less-than-rational AI, or even a poorly programmed AI writing your story.

There are a lot of quick and easy answers out there to your mind-body struggle that may be attractive in their simplicity. Maybe you've tried a lot of them? Do they leave you wanting something more substantial? The human mind-body dynamic is complex, but I've simplified the concepts into two simple human actions.

I've said them before, do you remember them?

Stand on your own two feet (Sensing Posture) and move forward (you'll learn this in the next chapter).

Separating Sensations and Emotions

It's key that you understand that sensing is distinct from your emotions. Let's be clear. Sensations are the experiences that arise and fall, and they are neutral—they last moments, not hours or days.

Emotions, on the other hand, can last longer and are personal. You assign meaning to a cluster of sensations. Psychiatrist Stanley Greenspan writes in *The Growth of the Mind* about the dual encoding of sensory experiences. We record both the physical properties of the sensory experience and the emotional qualities we connect to them. It's this early, pre-verbal process of encoding our emotions that lays down a scaffolding for cognition.

> *Thinking, therefore, requires two components [...] an emotional structure that sorts and organizes events and ideas even before we use words and symbols to represent them [...] Second, we need a process of testing, refining, or elaborating that then evaluates these thoughts in light of our capacity for logic [...] Viewing **intellect as based on emotion** [emphasis added] gives a new perspective on the process of learning to abstract.*[2]

Emotions are the foundation for our cognition because they direct action to test and refine our thinking, creating fundamental signals for taking one of two broad actions: do I move toward or away?

What you learn in this section will be a path to clear thinking that started with refining your sensing first. When you skillfully allow the neutral experience of sensing to arise and fall, you regain bandwidth that was

---

2 Greenspan et al., (1997). *Growth of the Mind*. Da Capo Press. p.26

previously consumed with merely holding things together. This increased capacity gives you the space for emotions to express honestly.

In life-or-death situations, we only have the bandwidth for action, powered by adrenaline. Emotions are put to the side until you find safety. That's why you'll see the outpouring of emotions once someone has been rescued from extreme peril. In safety, there is room to express authentic emotions.

As you develop refined sensory skills, your posture and movement will improve along the way. But ultimately, you are improving your capacity to pay attention and to discriminate, which is the solid platform your brain needs for clear thinking.

The aim of this section is to give you the tools for action that align with your intention, allowing you to do so with the whole of yourself. At the level of cognition, you can use your sensory perception and discrimination to give you space to feel your emotions while making clear choices. You can think with the whole of yourself (instead of cutting yourself off from feeling) because you are organizing your body to create the internal space you need.

Linking What You Feel to How You Behave

It's not a straight line from sensory cues to action. You're interpreting the imprint of body experience emotionally, assigning meaning to everything you feel. You're designed to do that, constantly seeking ways to categorize, evaluate, and interpret in order to understand, to form a narrative that makes sense, and on a very deep brain level, to conserve energy. So, while on the one hand, your body is trying to optimize posture (Sensing Posture), on the other hand, you take the shape that makes you feel safe and respond to how you believe you are seen in the world.

What your body needs to be upright and what your sense of self needs to feel safe and seen are different objectives but created during one unified, embodied process. Because the sensory body and emotional body are encoded together, making the distinction between a body sensory event, the meaning you place on it, and the beliefs you've built up about yourself over time is something you must consciously untangle.

Self-Control vs. Self-Regulation

Self-control is suppression to stop or prevent the body from doing what it's doing. It's a hierarchical approach that says, "top controls bottom."

Self-regulation is giving the body what it needs so it can do things better. It's a relational approach that says, "bottom informs top," and the conversation goes both ways. You learn self-regulation by understanding and responding to the body's needs. And you communicate with your own body through your Sensing Posture.

Self-control can be a necessary skill for certain situations and is often more about directing behavior in limited circumstances. This approach can be exhausting, however, when you rely on it for daily living. If you don't know how to align your internal experience with the actions you take, unmet needs that are lingering in your felt sense will ultimately catch up with you.

Self-regulation, on the other hand, is building a relationship with your body so you are collaborating with it in the sensory language it understands.

For example, perhaps your mother always told you to "stand up straight," so you consciously pull your shoulders back and stiffen your back to take the position. But it's exhausting, and you only do that when you feel like you need to be in performance mode, so the nagging will stop. Standing up straight is a chore and not an internal desire. You feel like a phony doing it and don't even know if you understand how to do it in a relaxed way.

Is there even an authentic way to stand up straight? Yes, through your Sensing Posture. You can find that internal desire to stand on your own two feet in a way that allows the front surface of your spine to support your head.

When a baby learns to stand and then walk, you see the innate delight. The baby is responding to an explosion of neurological connections. That feeling motivates the baby to explore, but with the internal feedback to find the right way to stay upright. What you've learned thus far is a return to the delight of that experience by paying attention to the body messages of safety, support, and power.

The capacity, the resilience, and the skill set to address these levels are collectively necessary because life happens, and it continues to happen, and you'll continue to be confronted with things that are difficult, surprising, and will throw you out of your body. When you learn new skills and build new resources, however, you can meet your unprocessed old experiences and unexpected new experiences from an expanded perspective.

To Summarize . . .

By accessing your sensing first, the stories that you tell yourself can change. Your Sensing Posture is your path to self-regulation because you are connecting fully to the nature of your sensory experience—one that is present moment, one that arises and falls.

On the front end of this journey, the learning curve might feel awkward because your daily movements are so familiar that it's weird to do them differently. But you'll quickly feel outcomes that make it worth the effort.

CHAPTER 6

Moving Forward with Intention

With the Sensing Posture, you learn to use your body as a resource through body organization. You balance the tension throughout your body using the 3 Keys so you can feel spacious and balanced, you engage the force of gravity using the Nautilus so you can feel empowered, and you enliven the connections within your core self through the Elastic Breath so you can feel your ease.

In this chapter, you'll learn what it takes to move forward. Overcoming old patterns requires more resources in your sensing. You can't change old patterns when you feel the same way. Your Sensing Posture is one way to expand your positive sensing experience.

Another way you can use your body as a resource lies in a pattern that lives in the design of your moving body. You can lean into it to find your way back to center. This pattern is the symbol of infinity. It loops between the left and right sides of your body. You'll find that it shows up in many other places in your body, but in this book, you'll learn how to find it in your pelvis. As you learn to feel it, you can leverage that innate pattern to return to your center again and again—predictably.

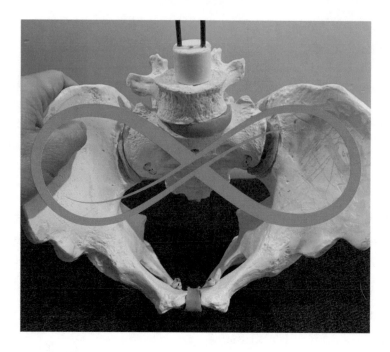

This repeated experience hones your trust in yourself to find your way back to center and to balance yourself out with the resources you will learn to access in an instant.

Movement is how we learn and understand our world. We move to discover, to understand. This is the prevailing understanding of brain function when it comes to conscious thought and action, according to leading neuroscientist Karl Friston.

"There's very little that you can do, apart from secretion, without movement, without your body . . . . The only way the brain can talk to the environment is through its body."[3]

In other words, you must move to learn about the world. You must take ac-

---

3   Friston, K. (2018, June 1). *Embodied Cognition Karl Friston* [Video]. Serious Science. https://www.youtube.com/watch?v=HW0JnjgCO3o

tion to test out your thoughts. If you consider moving your body as a way to **understand** the environment, does that change the way you consider how you might operate it? Remember, your body understands through sensing. Your movement is as much a process of learning how to feel as it is a process of executing or performing.

You're learning how to use the body to move in order to feel. To feel at ease, to feel connected, to feel your power, to feel centered, calm, and secure, to feel like the world makes sense. When you learn how to take actions that create these feelings, you can access your internal feelings of wholeness.

You learned how to feel connected and whole through your Sensing Posture in Steps A–C.

This next section helps you move forward with intention in Steps D–F.

> **Steps D–F are:**
>
> D. Metabolize old patterns.
>
> E. Take up all of your space.
>
> F. Make intentional choices.

Step D: Metabolize Old Patterns Using the Infinity Resolution Process

Walking is how humans move through the world, and it is unique from other species. We are the only species to walk this way on a regular basis. Occasionally, we find a gorilla or chimpanzee walking upright. Some even have this very human-like contralateral rotation in their spine as they walk. That means the upper and lower bodies swing in opposite rhythms. When one leg goes back, the arm on that same side goes forward, rotating the spine. Although some people lack this coordination (they walk in a homolateral pattern), we are designed to move with contralateral action.

In the Infinity Resolution Process, you identify and amplify that pattern through small movements, and then you deliberately create polarities (resource and difficulty) in your left and right sides so those opposites can balance each other out through the template of the infinity.

The internal bottom-up process of sensing is what psychiatrist and trauma expert Bruce Perry talks about when he's talking about empathy. Bottom-up processes that restore a sense of safety are necessary to build trust. The Sensing Posture builds safety, and the Infinity Resolution Process is the relational interaction within yourself between what's working and what's not.

VIDEO: INFINITY RESOLUTION PROCESS

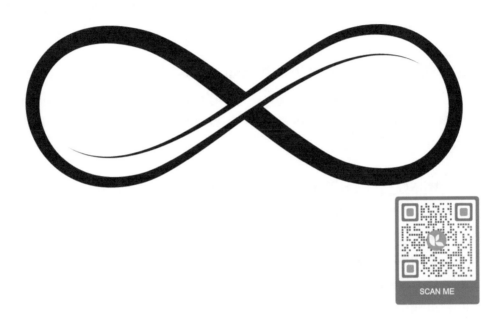

SCAN ME

Take 10 minutes here to watch the video. Make sure you can feel the infinity pattern within you. You spent the first 3 lessons developing your internal resources. In this phase, you are meeting your old patterns, and it will be natural to struggle a bit. When in doubt, reach for more resources.

How does that feel? Can you identify the infinity pattern that happens within your pelvis?

If you can't find it, don't worry, the pelvis holds a lot of patterning that can restrict you from getting this right away. You'll find it eventually.

If you feel this, you might recognize this internal movement as *push clouds* in chi gong or the internal pattern when you are skiing.

Can you bring that internal awareness into your walk? Just because you are walking does not mean you are using all the features available to you. We have a body that is designed with many redundant pathways for walking. If you feel back pain from going on a short walk, if you feel tired from long walks, if your feet hurt after walks, then you will love how you feel from accessing the fundamental internal movement of your walking pattern, the Infinity.

WHAT IT IS IN THE BODY: The human body, when walking, translates weight from one side to the other through the sacrum. Being able to feel the nuance and clarity of this action is a rhythmic and predictable action that calms your brain.

THE MEANING YOUR BODY SENDS TO YOU WHEN YOU USE THIS: You are built to move forward with momentum. You are designed to return to your center. Your resources are there to help you metabolize your difficulties. When you distinguish the polarity of your left and right sides and weave them back together through movement, you remind yourself of your embodied blueprint for resolution.

More Details about the Infinity Resolution Process

The template of infinity in your body is your path to recovery, again and again. It can be a single-use solution to a single problem, but it's also a principle of movement that lives deeply in your body.

The infinity symbol is tracked in the pelvis through our contralateral movement. There is an oscillation from one side to the other through a center point. This essential movement pattern can be leveraged as a full-body template for trauma resolution. This is a template that we know well, and it returns to you the power you couldn't access when you were stuck in old patterns. The key is to clearly identify the left and right polarities in your body and then weave them back together. We are always creating our center again and again. When you understand this, you'll have flexibility, fluidity, and virtuoso skills to be responsive in the moment, whatever it brings.

In trauma resolution, there is an emphasis on titration. The patient is exposed to small doses of trauma-related stress with the objective of building tolerance to their traumatic memories. Attention is paid to the sensations they experience. But the more significant emphasis in this approach is to seek and amplify your embodied resources first before you touch into trauma. In this diagram, you always start with your resource.

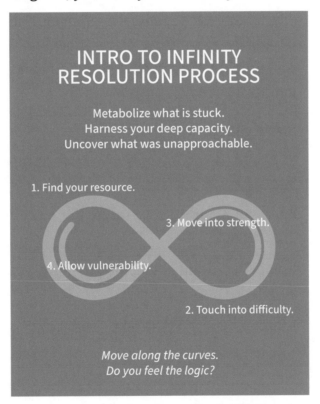

By oscillating through the infinity pattern from resource to difficulty, you can feel how to metabolize old patterns. You're training yourself to become familiar with and trust that predictable flow back to your center. To venture away from home and return is a process that you create again and again on different scales: a child reaches out to explore and runs back to momma when he is scared; a young woman leaves to explore the world and comes back to her hometown for a high school reunion; a refugee builds a new life in a new country and returns to taste the culture she had to leave behind, but she finds she is changed and no longer feels she can relate to her contemporaries who stayed because home is where she is now, who she is now. The resolution process returns to center, but just like walking, your center is moving forward.

Activating the Infinity

The Infinity is the template of resolution that is innate in your body's design. Before moving into the resolution process, you prepare your body first by priming its innate capacity to move forward.

Stand with your feet wider than your hips.

Roll onto the right edges of both feet, then roll onto the left edges of both feet.

Keep all your toes on the floor and stay in your Shin-Ankle.

Going back and forth, notice how your body turns as you do this.

Make sure you're not swinging your hips over to the side to do this.

Imagine that your torso is in a test tube and turning within the limits of that tube.

Look at a single point out in the distance.

Let the spine rotate under your steady head.

What do you feel? Where are you moving from?

If you imagine you are looking down into your pelvis, can you feel the movement along the infinity path?

It's a figure eight, and each loop traces its path deep in the hip sockets.

When you bank the turn in your right hip, notice the movement flow toward and across the midline.

It dives into the back of your left hip, banks the turn, and then flows toward and across the midline.

There's the infinity movement that you generate by just standing in place and turning.

If you've done chi gong, you might recognize this as very similar to push clouds movement.

You're reminding your body that it doesn't need to stay stuck, that it has internal mechanisms to keep flowing. When you lengthen on one side, unweight the other side, and transfer the weight, you move forward.

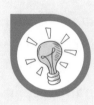

Using the Infinity for Resolution

We use that idea of flow and forward movement by encoding our body, our left and right sides, with what works and doesn't work for us.

This is the part where you use your intention to change things. You've activated the template of balance and resolution by tracking the infinity within you. Now you can use that template to create polarities in your left and right sides, so they can resolve in the center.

Sit and close your eyes.

Place your hands on your thighs.

Feel your hands touch the thighs, and feel your thighs touch your hands.

Designate the left hand as the resource hand.

Encode your left hand with a very specific moment, place, or thing that makes you feel expansive.

Make it specific and evocative so you can experience it now.

Include sensory details like the light, the sounds, the temperature, the smells.

Take a moment to feel the whole resourceful experience in your left hand. Your left hand represents this experience.

Designate the right hand as your challenge hand.

Encode your right hand with a very specific challenge.

Not a big thing like the entire relationship you have with your mother, but something specific.

Like how your stomach knots up when she asks a particular question.

Or what happens in your face when you hear a criticism that triggers you.

This is typically much easier to encode because it's constantly jumping into your consciousness to ask for our attention. You don't have to spend a lot of time encoding it.

Feel the difference between your left and right hands.

If you can't feel a difference, go back and embellish your resource hand.

You can embellish the memory with more sensory richness from your imagination—add the sounds of birds, brighten up the lighting, add fresh scents, generate sounds in your scene that you love to hear.

Make your perception of having resources become more alive in you.

Once you feel the difference between your left and right hands, alternate tapping your hands on each thigh.

Now let your mind go and allow your body intelligence to take over. Tap for 10–30 seconds.

Pause and feel the left and right sides.

Have they balanced out?

If not, continue tapping for 10 more seconds.

How do you feel now if you bring yourself to the challenge represented in your right hand?

If you still feel resistance, try again. Using more specific encoding, as if you are creating a scene in a film.

This resolution can happen very quickly, and it's not the intensity of the tapping or the duration of the tapping that makes it resolve. It's actually the setup. It's the way you enrich and amplify what's a resource for you so that it can overwhelm what you struggle with. When you back off and let the intelligence of your fast-acting subcortical brain take over you can rapidly resolve your challenge.

If it doesn't, then go back to encoding. Once you get more practice at encoding and amplifying what is resourceful for you, you'll find that this is a way that you can go through life. You're looking for what serves you. You're looking for what works.

And when you overwhelm your challenges with what works, then what is stuck in you starts to change. You start to metabolize it. You start to eat away at the edges. It starts to take away its insistent need to be addressed.

Sensing, Moving forward, and Brain Function

In your Sensing Posture, you work with body organization. A lot of that happens in your cerebellum. This part of the brain contains over three times more neurons than the rest of your brain. The right cerebellum controls the right side of the body for organization (as in the Sensing Posture).

The left somatic cortex (conscious movement brain) controls the right side of the body for movement.

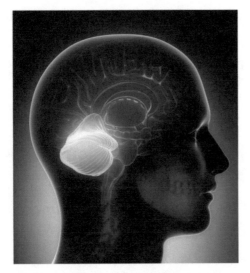

Right cerebellum

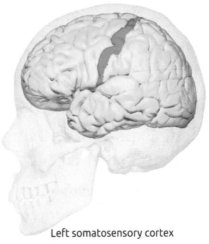

Left somatosensory cortex

*BodyParts3D, © The Database Center for Life Science licensed under CC Attribution-Share Alike 2.1 Japan.

Together, the right cerebellum and the left somatosensory cortex coordinate to control the right side of the body.

So the infinity pattern of movement connects the Sensing Posture (cerebellum for body organization of the same side) with the conscious movement body (somatic cortex for intentional movement of the body on the opposite side).

The Infinity Resolution Process is a specific process that I've seen work over and over again. The more skilled you get at practicing this, the more habitual it becomes, and the more you see how to apply it spontaneously when you feel yourself coming up against resistance or difficulty. You arm yourself with more resources in order to overcome obstacles so you can move ahead.

We go around all day with variable states. When something has become chronic, however, it hijacks our normal function. Sensations are impermanent by design. If something becomes chronic, a normally temporary experience becomes fixed into a context that includes beliefs, memories, and expectations. It can most definitely alter physiological processes, like the nociceptor sensitization that occurs in chronic pain or heavy scar tissue that appears after surgery, but it can also be dismantled with the right movement that organizes and stabilizes the body to its center.

Client Experience: Using the Infinity Resolution Process to Complete a Project

"I have been intending to tackle the big project of clearing the clutter and organizing my craft room for several years. Each break from work, the weeks passed, and nothing was accomplished.

This winter break, I felt an internal shift (not conscious). I started with creating a beautiful spot, stood and felt the feels—really letting it in. This became a motivator for the next step, standing back and feeling the accomplishment. Celebrating each step created resources within me. The night before I returned to work, I sat and realized I did it! I organized the whole room, including both closets.

I felt energy moving where in previous breaks I just felt depressed and stagnant. I can feel energy continuing to move. Not focusing on the problem (I have to tackle this job) but rather reaching for resources (the feeling of accomplishment and the feeling I got from beauty and organization) was a big key to this success."

Trauma in the Body

Are you dealing with an embodied trauma response? Embodied trauma is a response caused by an overwhelming experience you cannot process at the moment because you did not have the skill, time, or support to process and regulate.

Are you working with a trauma therapist? This method is not a replacement for professional psychological help. If you are working with a therapist or need one, please continue on the path. This work complements the psychotherapeutic process.

The process of working through trauma in the body starts with first building body resources with the Sensing Posture. When you work with your body to connect and be renewed by forces larger than you (such as the feeling of gravity), you are generating the experience of safety. Instead of trying to directly dismantle an embodied freeze response, you connect to the power of gravity through the language of movement. This sets up a context that makes sense to the body, paving an opening to metabolize old patterns through movement and oscillation.

An embodied freeze response is a body that tightens in response to stretching. It rebounds—sometimes with spasms—in response to a relaxation technique, and it might tremor instead of relax. Fighting a body in this state into relaxation is futile. It needs to feel safe, not be forced to let go. Easing your body into a deeply relaxed state without a strategy for integrating the changed state back into your normal daily life does not progress you. A traumatized body first requires experiences of connection before resolution can happen. That's why we start with building resources as the starting point.

In this process, you only work in therapeutic doses of exposure to triggers. As psychiatrist and trauma expert Bruce Perry explains:

> *Think about how you've handled difficulty in your own life. With*
> *things that are very hard to deal with, you don't want to talk about*

*the pain or loss or fear for forty-five minutes nonstop. You want to talk with a really good friend for maybe two or three minutes about some aspect of it. When it gets too painful, you step back, you want to be distracted. And maybe you want to talk more later on. **It is the therapeutic dosing that leads to real healing. Moments. Fully present, powerful, and brief** [emphasis added].*[4]

You will learn how to set yourself up to metabolize the rigid body patterns of trauma by alternating between resources and difficulty. When you are working with trauma triggers in your body, sometimes you don't even know where they come from. That is often the nature of somaticized trauma. Understanding how it fits into the narrative may take time to fall into place or may never be revealed if cognitive processing isn't necessary.

By working with your Sensing Posture, you are able to dip into moments of safety readily and frequently. By finding your internal template of resolution in the infinity pattern, you witness how polarities return to center again and again.

Your pelvis is a convergence of many things: your sense of self-support, your capacity to regulate your toilet habits, your center of sexual intimacy. Powerful patterns that have worked for decades to keep you together, however imperfectly, can't be dismantled unless you give your body other choices. The Infinity Resolution Pattern is a pattern of continual movement, an invitation to predictable and safe change.

Step E: Take Up Your Space Using Elongation

Once you find new openings in your body, you need to expand into those new spaces. Because you are not habituated to taking up this space, you

---

4 Perry, B. (2021) et al., *What Happened To You? Conversations On Trauma, Resilience, and Healing*. Flatiron Books. p.#113-#114.

will revert back to your old posture if you do not deliberately move in.

VIDEO: ELONGATION

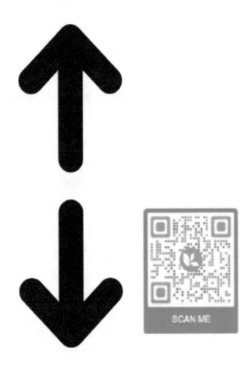

This video of the half-body stretch gives you the feeling of elongating your spine upwards and downwards at once. It's a very simple and powerful exercise that you can use quickly to establish access to your deep support.

WHAT IT IS IN THE BODY: After you've rebalanced your whole fascial webbing, you can deliberately expand into the new spaces you've created.

THE MEANING YOUR BODY SENDS TO YOU WHEN YOU USE THIS: The message here is to inhabit the fullness of your body, to take up all of the space you are capable of filling. You are showing up with the whole of yourself.

With the half-body stretch, you stretch the left side of the body to find how elongating one side of the spine facilitates the translation of movement to the other side and vice versa. You are distinguishing the polarities of your body and highlighting how the translation from side to side happens through the sacrum.

This alternating relationship between body halves reinforces the alternating pattern of the Infinity Resolution Process.

Activating Elongation through the Half-Body Stretch

Elongation is the process of dynamically inhabiting all of your spine in an expansive way. The half-body stretch is a quick way to remind yourself of the nature of expanding along one side of your spine that also naturally creates a slight contraction on the other side of your spine. In the full walking dynamics, it is a rotational action, but for ease of learning elongation, experience it on one side at a time.

Think of dividing the body into left and right halves.

Push down through the left foot and up through the left arm.

Stretch up and down along the side of the spine, staying in the Shin-Ankle.

As you do that, your opposite waist will shorten, unweighting the right foot.

That happens because the Sacral Key translates the movement through the pelvis and, in doing so, moves like this.

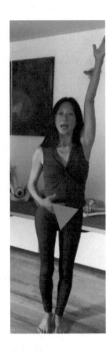
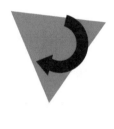

You are activating the connection of one side to the other through the translation of movement through the Sacral Key. Lengthening on the left side shortens the waist on the right, unweighting the right foot. This is the connection that happens in the walking step.

Try it on the other side.

As you reach, make sure you don't use your back muscles to go into extension.

Reaching up through the arm and down through the leg connects to the diaphragm.

Find your internal stretch, at the side surface of the spine, without leaning over to the side.

Look for a taffy-like stretch, where there's no hard stop at the end, like it's an infinite stretch.

You can do it first thing in the morning, lying down in bed.

You can do this sitting in a chair.

Step F: Make Intentional Choices Modeled by Your Visual System

Take this segment slowly. Attention training is full-brain training. You are working with a mental process as it's linked to your visual system. You'll be making a conscious choice. Look for sensory feedback such as watering or tearing in your eyes, relaxation around your eyes, or a feeling of mental clarity. Sometimes you may have a big shift, and your vision may cloud up for just a moment before it shifts into a new level of clarity.

VIDEO: MAKING CHOICES

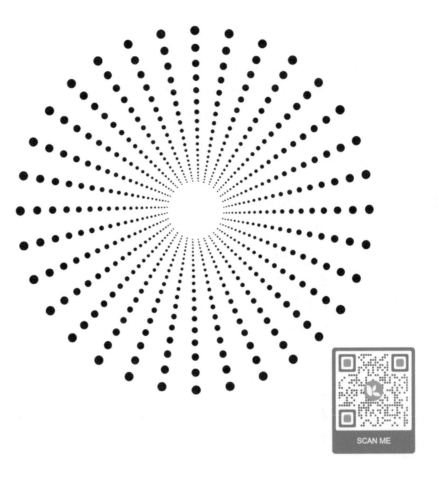

In this video, you'll experience how you can deliberately use your vision according to its innate design. This is one way to use a sensory foundation to help make a clear choice.

<u>WHAT IT IS IN THE BODY:</u> When you stimulate your peripheral visual system in this way, your visual perception focuses more easily on what you choose. You'll see with more clarity, more color saturation, or perceive

more movement in your peripheral vision.

There are almost twenty times more rods than cones in your retina, and the rods register movement, contrast, and shades of gray. Through this practice, you are stimulating these predominant structures in your retina.

When you think of peripheral vision, do you think that means the far outer edges of your visual field? It's actually everything that is not focal, which includes a lot. It's everything that is between you and the point of your focus, as well as what's beyond the point of your focus. Your visual focal point is a point in space that you choose, and everything else is what you *unchoose*.

THE MEANING YOUR BODY SENDS TO YOU WHEN YOU USE THIS: By doing this exercise, you'll get some insight into how to deal with the unknown. You are giving permission to your peripheral system to operate the way it was meant to operate—in motion and indistinctly. You are not trying to make clear what is not meant to be clear. You are not trying to focus on too much at any given moment.

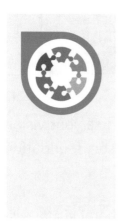

Activating Your Peripheral Vision by Making a Choice

Intention is what moves you forward. In fact, clear intention pulls you forward. Tunnel vision, on the other hand, blocks out everything that is still part of vision. This exercise teaches you that intention, like your focal vision, means unchoosing everything else.

Place your 2 index fingers out in front of you and look at the right fingertip.

As you look at this fingertip, notice that the other fingertip is in your visual field, but you can't see as much detail.

As you look at your right fingertip, see the wrinkles in that finger.

Look at the nail bed, see the little half-moon in your nail.

You can't see those on the left finger.

To prove that, move your gaze to look at the left finger tip.

Notice all the details that you previously did not see when you were looking at the right.

Pick out all the details that you see in the left finger.

You see the right with your peripheral vision.

It's there, but it's indistinct.

The right finger does not have the level of detail as the left, the one you're looking at.

Now go back to the right finger and notice the details you previously could not see with your peripheral vision.

What we're practicing here is observing the nature of deliberately choosing. To let something exist in the peripheral and not see it distinctly is how your peripheral vision works. Give yourself permission to notice something but let it be indistinct to relieve your visual system. You cannot see everything clearly all at once. That is a combination of memory and expectation. Your visual system only sees clearly in the moment the small point on which you focus. And it is easier to focus when you allow what is peripheral to be indistinct.

You see clearly where you choose to look, not where you used to look or where you want to look. To choose is to unchoose everything else. Because when you make a choice, you are with the finger that you're looking at, and you are deliberately not with the other finger. The other finger has a certain quality to it, which is indistinct but equally valid. What is unchosen is the field of possibility. You make something from this field become focal when you choose it, as demonstrated here by your visual system.

But as explained in this book, your choice is integrated with the whole of you. Your visual system is designed to only see one spot very clearly, and everything else that you're not focused on is indistinct. If you can get that into your thinking, you start to get clear with what it means to make a real choice—to commit with the whole of your sensing self and to move forward with the trust that you are designed to return to equilibrium.

After doing this exercise, what new things do you notice in your environment?

Another Visual Focus Experience

Now extend this exercise to allow the whole of the room to be indistinct as you focus on one finger. You'll see more clearly that everything except what you are focused on is actually indistinct.

Move around the room and notice how everything indistinct moves. But it moves with you as if everything is an extension of you. When you move, everything except what you choose to focus on is moving.

When you experience motion in your peripheral field in this way, by seeing movement as an extension of your own movement, you are in relationship to it. It's not separate from you.

How does noticing so much movement make you feel? And how do you feel about the point you chose to see clearly?

Many people do not use their peripheral vision. They don't actually see movement because observing too much movement produces anxiety. Often, they rely on the immediate memory of something instead of perceiving the movement as it happens. By design, your peripheral vision signals alarm in response to movement that is close to you and unexpected. It's a protective feature. But when inanimate objects are not moving, or when objects are moving in a predictable manner that is directly related to your own movement, you can release your peripheral system to register the awareness it was meant to. The safety of seeing movement that you control is acceptable, but the perception that movement is destabilizing because it's outside of your control can make you narrow what you perceive.

When you liberate your peripheral vision, you're also unburdening your focal vision from trying to make everything clear all at once. You're giving your visual system the opportunity to see more precisely by using more peripheral awareness (deliberate attention to movement and indistinctness).

How does it feel to understand that you don't create clarity with more focus but let it emerge with more attention to everything else? It sounds counter-intuitive, right? But it's the way your visual system works.

Using your visual system in this way connects your mental experience to the sensory impact you've generated through your Sensing Posture, through how you resolve difficulty, and how you take up space. A profoundly different posture and way of moving can feel strange compared to the familiar and protective shape that you've come to identify as you. To be able to make a choice in a way that aligns with your sensory system helps you organize your visual perception and mental process with your body sensing.

Vision and Choice

When you use vision as a proxy for clarity in intention, you invite a sensory process to undermine old patterns.

Here's my interpretation of what's happening: this way of using your vision is coordinating your brain. You're using the focusing capacity of your conscious thinking brain to overcome the energy-saving function in your lower brain. What does it take to convince the lower brain that change is worth the energy expenditure? Your lower brain processes much faster than your conscious, thinking brain. So it gets to an answer much more quickly than your thoughts. Can you even use your thoughts to change old patterns? I'm suggesting that when you concentrate your intention in the same way you allow your focal vision to emerge from the indistinct peripheral, you can.

How might you use this in daily life? To me, this is about making choices. My definition of anxiety is **the body's desire to do something and the heart's fear of choosing.** You can use this visual process to make choices that align with the whole of yourself. By clearly connecting to something, you perceive more dimensions of it. It doesn't mean everything else is ignored. You just put everything else into a category that is indistinct while you bring your attention to the one thing you choose.

Choosing in this way is a full commitment, but one that doesn't restrict you from making a different choice in the next moment. It does restrict you, however, from forcing yourself to try to see everything all at once or from going into tunnel vision in order to choose just one thing. When you truly choose, you choose one thing and give yourself permission for everything else to exist in a state that isn't totally clear.

Observing vs. Perceiving

The information we gather visually can be dissected into what we observe and what we perceive (i.e., interpret). Amy Herman is a lawyer and art historian who uses art to train people in law enforcement how to discriminate between observation and perception. By observing the matter-of-fact and mundane details that we might normally neglect to identify, we can move past biases and interpretations that distort what we think we see.

Betty Edwards' famous book and coursework *Drawing on the Right Side of the Brain* demonstrates how we can draw remarkably well when we move out of our interpretations and into our direct observation of what is actually in front of us. Let's say you are asked to draw a cat. Most people draw what looks like a cartoon image of a cat. They draw the representation of an abstraction they mentally identify as a *cat*. But say you turn the image of the cat upside down and cover it with paper, so you only see the top 10th of the image, and you draw to replicate only what you see, and then repeat that ten times. When you finish, you'll see that you've created a more accurate drawing.

Your Sensing Posture likewise trains you in direct observation. You observe the needs of your whole physical self without the abstraction of your identity self. The clarity of sensing in this way trains you to be anchored in the present.

Awareness, Attention, and Intention

I like to think of awareness as the ambient light, attention as the spotlight, and intention as the laser beam. Awareness is what you develop with the

Sensing Posture. It's the ambient light. Attention is using a spotlight to direct your energy toward a project—overcoming one emotional block, for example. But intention is the laser beam that draws out the creative manifestation of your thoughts by refining how you perceive the path forward.

How you perceive with intention (for pattern recognition, focus, and in alignment with your visual function) and how you listen so you can feel with the whole of yourself brings together the top-down thinking with bottom-up sensing.

Pattern recognition requires that you have some mechanism to look at yourself. You can do it in so many ways, and you do it so you can separate your observation of yourself from the action of yourself. You can do this through things like journaling, art therapy, or some process where your intention is to gain greater insight into yourself. But the most impactful part of your behavior is how you move through and interact with the world. You understand the world by testing it out. So as Karl Friston noted, you have to move through the world to understand.

To Summarize . . .

How do you feel? All six lessons can be used on their own but are more powerful when layered together. That'll come over time.

But to start right now, simply use what helps you feel better in your body. Build a resourceful body, one that sends you messages of support, power, and ease through your Sensing Posture. Practice reaching for those resources as you meet little challenges throughout your day.

With a resourced body, moving ahead becomes more than a mere walk.

☞ Seek out the infinity template of resolution whenever you're taking a walk.

☞ Take up your space to inhabit your new body by feeling how the half-body stretch happens in walking.

☞ Make a clear choice to connect with a point in the distance and feel how this connection can pull you forward as everything else moves in reference to you.

If you can bring the 3 Keys, Nautilus, and Elastic Breath into your life, you have accomplished a lot to restructure your body. Your awareness of your wholeness and internal connections improve how you move in daily life and in your physical activities.

If you can use the infinity template for resolution and take up your space through elongation, you are relieving your entire system of unnecessary holding. Your attention at this level of change allows you to feel your power and deliberately face difficulties with new resources.

And if you can change how to listen with your whole self while seeing with clarity, you can change the way you make choices through clear intention. When your actions align with your intention, the internal conflict that holds you back fades into the background, and you follow through on the commitments you make to yourself.

What you've learned here is a big agenda. It asks you to shift your efforts away from the feeling of pushing and working hard. Instead, you're being asked to put your effort toward paying attention in a new way—but only after you've reached for your resources first. Changing your perceptual habits can feel unusual in the beginning, but that will change as your whole body and mind open to your body's essential processing of gravity, light, and sound.

CHAPTER 7

How It All Comes Together

To break out of old patterns, it helps to understand how the body perceives things for different purposes: body organization, emotional content, and thinking.

How You Experience Your Body at Three Levels

The body at the *organizational level* is sensing. Sensations arise and fall. They are neutral and are designed to adapt. For example, you will smell burned toast when you enter a room, but after some time, you adapt and no longer notice the smell. Let's call this the bottom-up level.

The body at the *thinking level* is abstracted into words for communication, planning action, and contextualizing experiences. Words like *happy, joy, pleasure, fun, and home* are all examples of experiences that can feel different in each of us. These concepts are not single experiences but a set of experiences that come together to form beliefs. Beliefs serve many purposes, like belonging and self-identification. Let's call this the top-down level.

In between these two levels is the *emotional content level*, where we form meaning. We interpret bottom-up signals and can attribute negative or positive feelings toward those sensations. We contextualize and associate sensations with meaning based on our circumstances and personal capacities of awareness, attention, and intention. At this level, it's as if we take the present-moment experiences of sensory impressions and process them across time so we can recall and connect with the past, imagine and plan for the future, and creatively change the present.

This middle layer is why this book exists, so you can learn how to intentionally align the bottom-up neutral sensory experiences with top-down concepts of yourself and your world. You can choose how to morph this present moment with your intentional actions to suit the arc of your life story.

How does a person create meaning from experience? How do you metabolize patterns that have been keeping you stuck? How do you integrate big, transformative experiences back into your daily life? What is stopping you from doing the things you want to do? How do you stop doing the things you no longer want to do? What's preventing you from showing up the way you want to show up in your life?

What you learned in this book are the principles and basic embodiment skills to help you address those questions. The body skills integrate into mental abstractions that are both meaningful and make sense, so you can find the flow and break through what's stuck.

By now, you understand that this process is rooted in the intelligence of the sensory body. By working with the body first, we tap into a deep reservoir of evolutionary intelligence encoded in our bodies, accessible to our conscious perception.

Some models of the brain talk about the reptilian brain or primitive brain in a dismissive way. This model of the brain implies this: the cortex is the newest part of the brain, the smartest part of the brain, and needs to be in charge of this unruly primitive, more ancient brain.

Here's another way of looking at it. The evolutionary intelligence deep in our bodies has the wisdom to make quick decisions, and to process based on millions of years of data, while the young part of our brain takes much more time to figure something out. This wiser brain processes data millions of times faster than the young cortex. Over millions of years, this deep brain has learned how to stand and walk. Of course, this deep brain shouldn't be in charge of something like problem-solving when someone hacks into your bank account. But this deep brain holds down the fort, so you don't have to worry about eating right now or in the next ten hours until you resolve the danger of losing control of your finances.

When the evolutionarily young brain—the revered neocortex—is overwhelmed, it can't make sense of what is happening. The deep brain freezes the moment until your young brain is better equipped to process and make sense—until your young brain gains wisdom. It's able to do this with more data, more life experiences, and more learned skills. And then, it can transmute direct experiences toward resolution and growth.

When you build up your embodied resources first, this expanded capacity will offset the cascade of embodied feelings that can completely disorient you when you bump up against old trauma. If you learn to discover, generate, and access resources in a variety of ways, you'll develop a wellspring of support to meet old challenges.

The goal is to make the act of connecting to resources a spontaneous and normal part of your life. Those things that are resourceful to you are the experiences, memories, and connections that make you feel expansive, joyful, optimistic, and confident. These embodied resources will help you overwhelm and metabolize the old restrictions that currently limit you.

Intention and Information Overwhelm

This concept of choosing, as I illustrate through your visual system, is a critical skill when faced with uncertain or incomplete information. This is the case in most circumstances—there is more than one way to see something.

Optical illusions illustrate this concept nicely. In the spinning dancer illusion by Nobuyuki Kayahara, the totality of information to determine the direction of spin is ambiguous. There are not enough conclusive signals to indicate which way she is spinning. So your brain has to make a choice. And sometimes, she flips, and sometimes she doesn't.

You can influence that choice consciously if you know what to look for and how to make a choice with your whole body. Use what you know about your body and see if you can deliberately make her flip. I'll let you try it first before offering a hint.

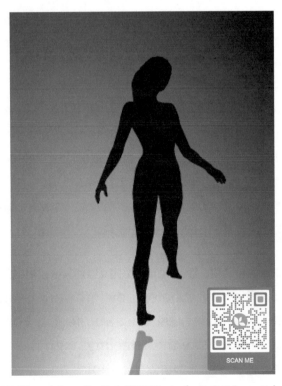

Copyright (C) 2018 Neuroinformatics Unit, RIKEN Center for Brain Science, Nobuyuki Kayahara

Hint: use mirror neurons so your body mirrors hers. Experiment and use your head position, your eye position, your spinal position, your arm, and your leg. Found something that works consistently? Head position, especially leaning back a bit, is a powerful cue.

But imagine you can't find a way to predictably flip her.

I'll tell you a story to explain it. I say this is a test of brain dominance. If you are right-brained, she spins clockwise, and if you are left-brained—the opposite. Innocuous, no big deal. But say you decide you are left-brain dominant, and I tell you left-brain dominant people are more likely to develop dementia. And that my luxury brain cure weekend retreat will fix that.

There is a slippery slope of belief that rests on the desperation for simple solutions to complex issues. Sometimes it makes sense to slide down that hill a few times because you're in the gathering data phase. But other times, you're just driving yourself through the same failed journeys again and again because your pattern is this: failing to commit to yourself in the choices you make.

I believe it's useful to give space in our beliefs for all the things we can't understand because having certainty can limit our discoveries. However, failing to test beliefs or commit to a direction can also limit capacity for growth. Definitive ideas on the nature of what you are doing are, in fact, only a deliberate choice because the reality is usually ambiguous. And in ambiguity, choices can be made FOR you or BY you.

What you've learned in this book is to find more signals of trust in yourself and a way to bring your whole body into your choices. Not because you know it all and not merely because you feel it. But because you can reliably and predictably create those feelings with the choices you make. When you know how, you can make the choice and flip the dancer at will.

That's a story that I'm giving you to explain how you can be more conscious in your perception, more present in your choices. I made a deliberate choice to work through the body because it serves as a feedback loop for internal alignment between sensing and intention.

How to Take Action When Faced with the Unknown

Taking the first step into the unknown requires a bit of courage. The Collins Dictionary defines courage as "the quality shown by someone who decides to do something difficult or dangerous, even though they may be afraid." The Latin root of the word courage is *cor*, which means *heart*. Courage is having the heart to take action, so consider that the first step into the unknown might require connecting to your heart.

When you are disheartened, you lose heart, you lose courage, and you lose the spirit to take action. How often do you allow yourself to follow your heart?

When I was studying yoga therapy in India at the Krishnamacharya Yoga Mandiram, I was also taking private Vedic chanting lessons. My teacher asked me if I understood the word *manas*. I replied, "Yes, it means mind," and I pointed to my head. She corrected me and placed her hand on her heart—*manas*.

Taking action with the fullness of yourself comes from this seat of the Sensing Posture. Training your attention to your Sensing Posture expands your direct experience of trust and stability, over and over again, during the mundane actions in your daily life. By creating a level of internal predictability, you have more room to feel from the heart instead of micromanaging your body from the thinking brain.

Where Are You Going?

Clients have often asked for more reading material to help them absorb what I was teaching and to help them construct a mental model of what they were feeling.

I created and refined this approach because I was always driven by one question:

> ### How can I teach people the principles and skills to feel calm and empowered so they can take useful action when they need it most?

Not just after a session. Not just when they came to see me. And not just when they did their exercises. You don't need more on your to-do list.

That mission has driven me to create what you've learned in this book. My goal is to teach you lessons so you can discover your thinking body in order to move beyond the old stories you tell yourself.

Where are you now? At your core, you are a product of your experiences. You can try to erase, run away, or even heal them. But you are unconsciously or consciously creating your life from those experiences. You actually have unused skills right now that you haven't fully accessed. In this book, you've learned an embodied way to access trust and belonging, how to process difficulty using the native design of the body, and how to move forward with intention.

This body approach enables you to consciously create from your experiences. to amplify your embodied resources to feel connection, safety, power, and ease so you can skillfully access your capacities.

CONCLUSION

*I*f you remember nothing else from this book, remember that there's a part of you that is bigger than yourself, and it is connected to the forces outside of you. When you find that and integrate it through your body through the Sensing Posture, you change the nature of how you organize your body. And when you move your body in order to feel, working with its innate design through the Infinity Resolution Process, you change your capacity to move forward.

Taking the time to learn this is a worthwhile investment. As philosopher Mark Johnson notes:

> *Coming to grips with your embodiment is one of the most profound philosophical tasks you will ever face. Acknowledging that every aspect of human being is grounded in specific forms of bodily engagement with an environment requires a far-reaching rethinking of who and what we are, in a way that is largely at odds with many of our inherited Western philosophical and religious traditions.*[5]

The first step you'll have to take is to try a video. Congratulate yourself on taking that step. Play around with remembering something from that video to use in your daily life. Integration into your daily life is the simplest way to make the change meaningful and impactful.

Then reread the section about that video. Let it sink into your mental model of yourself and your body.

---

5 Johnson, M. (2007) et al., *The Meaning of the Body: Aesthetics of Human Understanding*. University of Chicago Press. p.1.

Try another video. The concepts of this book are meant to be considered in conjunction with your direct embodied experience from using what you learn in those videos. And they are meant to be investigated over and over again, from different angles, until you find yourself automatically living in your Sensing Posture, using the Infinity Resolution Process as you walk and move through your blocks, increasing the clarity in your actions.

Reviewing What You've Learned

The overall process, as I described it in this book, consists of the following:

☞ Finding your Sensing Posture experience, which includes the meaning it sends your brain: stability, power, ease.

☞ Using your body template to move forward and change your story.

The six lessons in this process:

<u>Your Sensing Posture: Find calm, power, and ease</u>

A. 3 Keys

B. Nautilus

C. Elastic Breath

<u>Your Path Forward: Metabolize old patterns, take up your space, move forward with intention</u>

D. Infinity Resolution Process

E. Elongation

F. Making choices

Taking the First Step

This work is more complicated to read about than it is to feel results. The more you understand in your body, the more you will train yourself to seek more subtle and more personally meaningful outcomes and feel new results. Your discoveries will continue to unfold in ways you can't imagine right now.

The key is to take action and start the process—no matter how small.

To help you work through this book, you can receive bonuses when you sign up here:

https://www.coherentbody.com/when-things-stick-bonuses

What is the path from merely feeling safe to having the courage to move forward? For me, the one thing I needed to do was commit to myself, to come home to my body. That was the first step that enabled me to take the actual actions I needed in my life. I was able to reclaim myself when I found access to my embodied trust.

When I left my well-paid job working at a small company with smart people, I had very little clarity on what my life would look like. And very little assurance I was making the right choice. But I was sure I could not stay on the path I was on.

When your intention is on how you want to feel, the choice to stay the same comes off the table.

It's my hope that what you've learned here has given you concrete actions you can take to create, at a minimum, a shift in your body. Please apply these lessons as you would conduct an experiment, noticing where you are before using these skills and comparing where you are after.

How to Connect with My Team

I've carefully designed and tested what you've learned here to make outcomes as direct and immediate as possible. If you'd like more expansive help to guide you deeper, you can connect with my team to see if what I offer is a good fit for you. I offer a live coaching program where you'll get access to more videos as well as regular live group practice and coaching sessions. The value of going through this process with other people who are likewise committed is a powerful process and works as an accelerant to your process.

Book a complementary 15-minute consult to determine if our live coaching program can help you.

For more info

Schedule a consult at:

https://www.coherentbody.com/when-things-stick-consult

Contact: support@coherentbody.com

Helping Others

If you've found this book valuable, I would be so grateful if you gave a copy to someone who could benefit from it.

I want to offer special gratitude to the members who have worked online with me over the years and helped bring a new dimension to this body of work with their participation, enthusiasm, and openness.

ABOUT THE AUTHOR

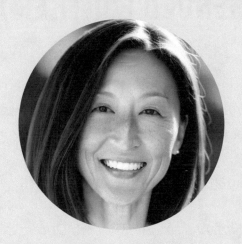

I'm a somatic movement teacher and bodyworker with over two decades of experience creating body solutions for clients. My goal has always been to help people make enduring and sustainable changes in their bodies that they can carry into their daily lives. Like most dedicated professionals who work with the body in this way, I am driven to understand how mental and emotional connections show up in the body. I'm particularly drawn to understanding how the deep currents of trauma distort a body.

My professional training includes yoga therapy at the Krishnamacharya Yoga Mandiram, Continuum Movement with Emilie Conrad, somatic movement with Hubert Godard, manual therapies in craniosacral, visceral manipulation, myofascial release, and perceptual training in the Tomatis Method™ sound therapy and natural vision. The work of psychiatrists, neuroscientists, and academics as they apply it to the sensory system has informed how I work with the body in movement.

RECOMMENDED FURTHER READING

Introduction to the developmental neurobiology of trauma:
What Happened to You? Conversations on Trauma, Resilience, and Healing
by Bruce D. Perry (psychiatrist and neuroscientist) with Oprah Winfrey

Emotions as a fundamental navigational system and the foundation for cognition:
The Growth of the Mind: And the Endangered Origins of Intelligence
by Stanley I. Greenspan (psychiatrist)

How sensory processing and attention regulate behavior:
A User's Guide to the Brain: Perception, Attention, and the Four Theatres of the Brain
by John J. Ratey (psychiatrist)

How meaning and purpose can liberate you:
The Will to Meaning: Foundations and Applications of Logotherapy
by Viktor E. Frankl (psychiatrist)

How meaning is encoded in our memories:
The Forgetting Machine: Memory, Perception, and the Jennifer Aniston Neuron
by Rodrigo Quian Quiroga (neurologist and physicist)

How sensations are perceived and interpreted in your neuroanatomy:
How Do You Feel? An Interoceptive Moment with Your Neurobiological Self
by A. D. Craig (neuroanatomist)

Stories of the brain's capacity to change:
The Brain's Way of Healing: Remarkable Discoveries and Recoveries from the Frontiers of Neuroplasticity
by Norman Doidge (psychiatrist)

How trauma is stored in the body:
The Body Keeps the Score: Brain, Mind, and Body in the Healing of Trauma
by Bessel van der Kolk (psychiatrist)

How the mind interprets experiences through the body:
The Embodied Mind: Cognitive Science and Human Experience
by Francisco J. Varela (biologist), Evan T. Thompson (philosopher), Eleanor Rosch (cognitive psychologist)

Mind, body, and consciousness:
The Meaning of the Body: Aesthetics of Human Understanding
by Mark Johnson (philosopher)

Emotional stress and disease:
When the Body Says No: Exploring the Stress-Disease Connection
by Gabor Maté M.D.

Suppressed rage and back pain:
The Mindbody Prescription: Healing the Body, Healing the Pain
by John E. Sarno M.D.

Made in United States
Troutdale, OR
02/19/2024

17826131R00073